Scholarly Pursuit of Nursing Science

Scholarly Pursuit of Nursing Science

One Nurse's Journey

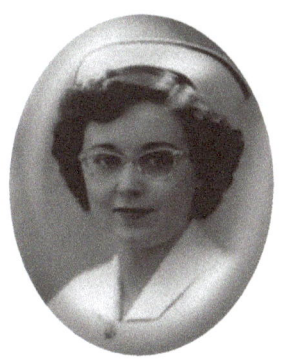

Floris Ethia King, Ph.D.

Professor Emeritus
A.T.C.M. Solo Piano Performer, University of Toronto
Reg. N. Toronto East General and Orthopedic Hospital
B.Sc. N. School of Nursing, University of Toronto
M.P.H. School of Public Health, University of Michigan
Ph.D. School of Public Health, University of North Carolina

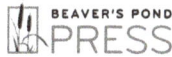

Scholarly Pursuit of Nursing Science © copyright 2013 by Floris Ethia King. All rights reserved. No part of this book may be reproduced in any form whatsoever, by photography or xerography or by any other means, by broadcast or transmission, by translation into any kind of language, nor by recording electronically or otherwise, without permission in writing from the author, except by a reviewer, who may quote brief passages in critical articles or reviews.

Any unique capitalization, punctuation, spelling, sentence structure, or grammatical choices found in this text are not flaws but are an integral part of this book, intentionally expressed and approved by the author, and meant to enhance the appeal of this independently produced work.

ISBN: 978-1-59298-959-1
Library of Congress Control Number: 2013917689

Printed in the United States of America
Book design by Mayfly Design and typeset in Arno Pro
First Printing: 2013

17 16 15 14 13   5 4 3 2 1

Beaver's Pond Press, Inc.
7108 Ohms Lane
Edina, Minnesota 55439
(952) 829-8818
www.BeaversPondPress.com

To order, visit www.BeaversPondBooks.com
or call (800) 901-3480. Reseller discounts available.

To the memory of my parents

Thomas King
1.4.1882 – 2.26.1966

Beatrice Maude King
9.20.1901 – 11.27.1986

Remembered with gratitude and love.

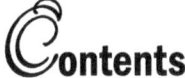
Contents

Foreword .... *xi*
Special Recognitions and Endorsements .... *xiii*
Prologue .... *xv*

CHAPTERS

ONE 1
Toronto East General and Orthopedic Hospital
1948–1952

TWO 7
University of Toronto School of Nursing
1952–1955

THREE 10
Public Health Nursing in Etobicoke, Ontario
1955–1958

FOUR 16
University of Michigan, School of Public Health, Ann Arbor, Michigan, USA
1958–1959

FIVE **18**

Study of Health Needs, Concerns, and Resources of 47 Counties of Ontario, Canada, Health Education Director, Ontario TB Association and within the Province of Ontario

1959–1964

PHOTOGRAPHIC INSERTS (19) **20**

SIX **30**

University of North Carolina, School of Public Health, Chapel Hill, North Carolina, Ph.D. Program

1964–1967

SEVEN **33**

Director of Programs, Nursing, Nursing Consultant, National TB and Thoracic Society, Ottawa, Canada

1967–1968

EIGHT **35**

University of British Columbia, Department of Nursing, Associate Professor, Director to Launch New Masters Program in Nursing, Vancouver, British Columbia, Canada

1968–1971

NINE **40**

Dalhousie University, School of Nursing, Halifax, Nova Scotia, Canada, Professor and Director of Nursing to Develop a Regional Masters Program in Nursing for the Maritimes

1971–1974

TEN **44**

Texas Woman's University, Denton, Texas, USA, Professor, Assistant Dean, and Director of Ph.D. in Nursing Program

1974–1975

ELEVEN **46**

University of Minnesota, School of Nursing, Minneapolis, Minnesota, USA, Professor, Associate Dean, Director of Graduate Program, Doctoral Program Proposal Grant Writer, and Director of Approval of Ph.D. in Nursing Program

1975–1991

Two Nurse Scholars, Lin and Lu, Spend a Research Quarter and Return with a Research Proposal in 1983

1982–1983

TWELVE **50**

Highlights of the Visit to the University of Kuopio, Finland

1985–1986

THIRTEEN **60**

Return to the University of Minnesota School of Nursing

1986–1991

FOURTEEN **62**

A Few Concluding Moments of Thought and Thank You

ARTICLES

ARTICLE #1 .... **67**

King, Floris Ph.D. 1971 First National Conference of Research in Nursing Practice, Ottawa, 1971 Department of National Health and Welfare. Grant Number 610-22-1xx

ARTICLE #2 .... **73**

The Formative Years of the Author, 1927-1948

APPENDIXES

APPENDIX A **81**

Nursing Model of Research Floris E. King Ph.D., 1972

APPENDIX B **83**

The elderly coping at home: a study of continuity of nursing care. Floris E. King, Professor and Research Officer, School of Nursing, University of Minnesota; Judy Figge RN Director and Chief Executive Officer, Austin Management Corporation; and Patricia Harman RN MS, Research Assistant Graduate Program in Nursing, University of Minnesota. Journal of Advanced Nursing, 1986, 11, 41–46 Accepted for publication 1 May, 1985.

EPILOGUE **97**

Foreword

When I receive a phone call asking for Jack, I know it is from a family member. Now, with years gone by, Floris is one of a few who calls me Jack.

Floris E. King, ATCM, RMT, BScN, MPH, Ph.D., has been a scholar and musician almost since the day she was born. Her commitment and the giving of herself to the growth and future development of nursing science, and the quality of nursing care has gained her recognition throughout Canada, the United States, and in Finland. It has been a bountiful commitment.

She is now retired and resides in Minneapolis, Minnesota, USA. Our family's theme song? "Keep in Touch."

—Judge John (Jack) Guy

Special Recognitions and Endorsements

I am convinced that each of us never reaches their full potential, but Floris has reached and achieved many milestones in an exceptional record of her Scholarly Pursuit of Nursing Science. A long journey of excellence from the time I sat with her in class lectures. CONGRATULATIONS!

—Jean Kennedy Campbell, former chairman, Centennial College of Applied Arts and Technology, Board of Governors

Floris showed her leadership early in our nursing careers. She formed a student nurses' choir. We sang at local churches. Her desire was to be top of her class.

—Helen McBrine, past chairman and life member, Hospital Auxiliary of Ontario Region #6

Having known Dr. King for almost six decades, I am not at all surprised by her accomplishments in academia. She is not only greatly motivated, but also a powerful motivator. She is an accomplished pianist and inspired me to reach heights I would never have attempted without her help and influence. Scholarly Pursuit of Nursing Science is a poignant and compelling diary of dedication to a preeminent purpose, a determination to finish the course set before her on a pathway of service and courage.

—Dorothy Moon, former neighbor, student, and a friend for life, Claremont, Florida

Echoes of the ART of nursing are audible as Floris King describes her journey in pursuit of the SCIENCE of nursing. Concern for patient/family needs is never

lost amid the theories and grants. This book may inspire others—in nursing and other professions—to capture and write their journey—stories.

—Carolyn Williams Ashburn, former nurse educator, hospital and hospice volunteer, part-time hospital staff chaplain

Dean S. Nelson, Ph.D., Dean of the School of Nursing, University of Toronto, flew to me August 2011 to present me with a special award. It is a medal award entitled Top Graduate of the School of Nursing, University of Toronto at the 90th Anniversary Celebration of the School of Nursing. I was overjoyed to learn it was a peer vote. And it was so lovely to meet, greet, and visit with Dean Nelson.

Prologue

This is simply a story of life happenings of a nurse as she went through growth periods in herself and in the nursing profession.

In nursing today there are so many opportunities to grow in scholarly knowledge and skill, as well as so many problems and concerns that need working out – including inter- and intra-disciplinary opportunities at home and abroad. There is so much to learn and do, and so many hands to reach out to – and it's all possible.

To continue the complexity of growth in both knowledge and skill, it is important to:

1. Provide continued opportunities and challenges for our nurse scholars in their own research/scholarship/leadership areas (with identifiable outcomes and actions);
2. Effect interdisciplinary support for health organizational studies on specified shared problems, concerns, and needs: (with identifiable outcomes and actions);
3. Support intra-disciplinary studies on shared problems, concerns, and needs: ex. With law, legal issues, child welfare, social work, etc. (with identifiable outcomes and actions);
4. Support intra-disciplinary nurse leadership studies with international agencies/groups/countries with related and shared concerns, problems, and needs (with identifiable outcomes and actions); and finally:

5. Support international nursing leadership research for continued knowledge growth and understanding of all countries' needs and nursing's leadership skills. Priorities will need to be set, the establishment of which I have every confidence in our present leadership. One of the riches of our nursing profession is the evolvement of highly qualified nurse leaders. These leaders have facilitated growth and creativity in clinical and community settings as well as explored and further developed the expansion of scholarly education.
6. It has been an exciting privilege to be a part of this growth period, as well as share in the continuing evolution of enriched nursing care, education, and research.
7. There have been a wide variety of challenges and exciting occurrences, many of which I will now recount. The past is not static. Every memory that comes back is a gift, and one fully realizes the importance of these experiences as the years go by.

There's a poem I would like to share with you. I have carried it in my wallet for some 40 years.

Bridge Builders

"The weary traveler on a lone highway
Came at the evening, cold and gray
To a chasm vast and deep and wide.
The traveler crossed in the twilight dim;
The sullen stream had no fear for him,
But he turned when safe on the other side
And built a bridge to span the tide.
Kind friend, said a fellow traveler near,
You are wasting your strength in building it here,
Your journey will end with the ending of day,
You never again will pass this way;
You have crossed the chasm vast and wide,
Why build a bridge at eventide?
The traveler lifted his old gray head;
Kind friend, in the path I have come he said
There follows after me today a youth
Whose feet will pass this way;
This chasm which has been as naught to me
To that youth may a pitfall be.
He too must cross in the twilight dim.
Kind Friend, I am building the bridge for him."

—WILL ALLEN DROMGROOLE, 1934

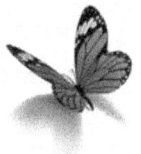

ONE

Toronto East General and Orthopedic Hospital

1948 – 1952

After many prayers and much thought, visits and discussion, I decided to enter the nursing profession. In the fall of 1948, I entered the Toronto East General and Orthopedic Hospital. Having spent my early years - very early years - as a concert pianist, I saw and felt the concerns and anxieties of many audiences, individual musicians and community groups at the close of the Second World War.

In music, musicians study not only the form, structure, and intonations of the music selection, but also the composer's life, the political, social, and economic factors that could have affected the composer's being and sensitivity. This helps the musician (me) to "intune" with the composer by understanding the time each particular piece was written. Basically, these elements are a reflection of the composer musician's essence of being. A concert pianist must also learn the formality of conduct on the stage, called stage presence. In order for me to learn this, the famous Canadian pianist Mona Bates had me take opera and Italian classes. However, the one with whom this experience was "endured" was my professor's very large police dog! He checked my every move as he sat under the grand piano – and it was obvious he was not fond of my singing. I also think he knew I was terrified of him – and didn't much like him either! We both survived the experience!

Although it is difficult to transpose intuning into nursing, a certain protocol is also called for in procedures in the delivery of care. For patient care it is essential. Nursing was a complete change of life for me. Up at 6:00 in the morning, prayers and breakfast at 6:30 and on duty on your floor by 7:00. We worked 7 to 7 day shifts, six days a week, with 2 hours off in the afternoon; Sunday afternoons we had 5 hours off and 7 to 7 night shifts with 2 hours off some time after midnight.

All the nursing students stayed in a big dormitory. My roommate, Eine Ronty, was very special, and we were fortunate to have our days and nights coincide. Not all did.

We started with lectures and personal care and procedure demonstrations. Within three months we were "on the floor." It was so great being with OUR patients. We didn't have all the mechanical equipment that is available today, but an IV was enough of a challenge then. There were difficult moments, of course.

Morendo

A woman died tonite,
I was down the hall,
The Special with her didn't care –
She didn't care at all.

I helped to turn her once,
How wonderful she was,
She tried to help and even smiled,
How lovely she was.
The husband stood by her,
Her Mother too was there –
You'll look after all the children Joe,
Her children were her only care.

Her abdomen was so taut,
Her breathing short and quick,
The doctor said they'd done all they could –
She was just too sick.

A lady died tonite,
I was down the hall,
The nurse with her didn't care –
She didn't care at all –

—FLORIS E. KING, 1949

We felt our uniforms were special – pink, short sleeved tops with the rest of the uniform white, bibs, aprons, short sleeved cuffs and leather shoes and stockings. After our preliminary preparation, we received our caps at the capping ceremony – what a delight. Of course we had to wait until we graduated to wear a black band on our caps; they were a prized symbol of accomplishment at that time.

I would like to see nurses in some form of uniform today – if only to help patients distinguish between a nurse and a cleaning lady. It also gives the nurse a sense of pride. Interns have their short white jackets, and the doctors have long white coats (except those in surgical greens or blues, but you know they are just out of surgery). Okay well, just a thought. I am thankful I experienced the pride of a nurse's uniform.

The schedule of our experiences was a rotation through the hospital wards: medicine, surgery, maternity, orthopedics, emergency and operating rooms. First we would be circulating nurses and then scrub nurses. Then there was the child care experience I had at Sick Children's Hospital, down on University Avenue. It was a top-notch hospital. One remarkable experience I had there was when I was the only nurse on 7 to 7 in the post-surgical ward. I loved it – giving the children their night care, comforting them, and yes, I even sang softly to them. The night supervisor made her rounds twice a night - unless there were emergency admissions. At 7:30 to 8:00 p.m., I would at times quietly sing, which settled the little ones to sleep.

A most difficult experience for me was in the Premature Nursery – such tiny, sick little ones, with IV in a blood vessel on their scalp. Counting those drops and second by second monitoring was a very tense moment for me. I talked softly to them, stroked them gently and hummed songs quietly to them. You could actually feel the dear ones relax.

You will not be surprised to learn that, yes, I started a student nurses' choir. It was a challenge to work in the time for practice - but we all did it.

We sang for the Sunday evening services in most of the large and medium sized churches in Toronto. We were well recognized in our uniforms! Here come the nurses! Jean Kennedy, one of our choir nurses, wrote me a note to say how much the church groups she had heard from enjoyed us. Jeannie was a special pal to all of us. Actually, all of our class were tops. Helen McBrien still organizes a yearly outing for us all. I've been too ill to go lately, but I love to learn about each and every one. They continue to be special.

The Toronto Monday morning papers carried large pictures and stories about the hospital's Student Nurses' Choir and that we sang in our pink and white uniforms. I had the choir learn anthems (including tenor – no bass!), and we all enjoyed it so much. I learned later that the doctors at the hospital got together and charted buses for us to get to the 7 p.m. services on time. With 7 to 7 duty, our choir nurses took their two hours off at 6 p.m. so they could change into clean uniforms! The buses returned us to the student residence after the service. I wondered if Mona Bates saw the Monday morning papers – I hope so! I know Mother did. I thought they might write me a note after I stopped concert piano, but I never heard from them. I would have liked to keep in touch with them.

Because of becoming so well known, our Nurses' Choir was invited to sing at the Toronto Star Free Concert, which was held yearly for invited choirs. We sang in our uniforms, of course, and when we "swung" "Bones, dem Bones." The whole audience responded with glee. After that, one of the top choir directors in the city came looking for me. I stayed at the back, but Jean Wallace Spalding (Instructor of Nursing) pushed me forward – and there I was! He said, "You're the choir conductor? Tell me, whose arrangement did you use for 'Bones'?"

I said, "Oh! That was mine." You should have seen the surprise on his face. I was quietly pleased. I thought, *As so often happens, music will bring people together* – it does it again!

While still keeping a toe in musical waters with the choir, I went from one ward to another, taking more responsibility as time passed. One of my patients I shall never forget. I cared for her during the night. She was the sweetest elderly soul. Her favourite saying was: "Now isn't that just too bad!"

Aime: 3:15 a.m.

Oh Aime, my Aime – oh there you go –
Here – pull on this – not the rope – Oh No –
It's 3:15 and time you slept –
Let's settle down – No, not yet?
Here, let's have a drink of this nice hot tea –
Oh Aime – now look – it's all over me,
The bed is wet – let's change it again
Up and over, back this way – I'll never be the same-
There – now it's past time for sleep
You've had enough luminal to last you a week,
Oh, at last, asleep – what peaceful repose –
Left leg cocked high – now touching her nose.
Oh Aime, our Aime – we do love you, you know
From your wee growth of whiskers right down to your toes.
At times you're so naughty, to give you away we might be glad –
But then your sauciness always wins us:
"Now, isn't that just too bad!"

—Floris E. King

The choir sang for the last time at graduation, 1951.

*I did not finish until 1952 because I had to make up time for illnesses and a bad bout of pneumonia.

Being a Nurse

Throughout this life
Our task is great
Our very lives
To make or break.

We each must strive
Our destiny to build –
Thru Faith and Love,
Strength and Will.

A nurse must grow
In herself and her skill –
Without both you see
Each would be nil.

But a nurse's life
Is more difficult to tell –
Not only herself must grow,
But her patients - as well.
A formidable task
You shout in accord?
But no closer way
Of serving the Lord.

—Floris E. King, 1951

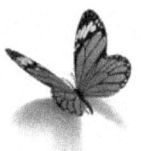

TWO

University of Toronto School of Nursing

1952 - 1955

After a lovely, long summer rest, I eagerly launched into academic life.

I decided to specialize in public health nursing. Now I could start fulfilling my dream – helping individuals, families, and working with communities. I thought, *Wonderful! And the programme at U of T is excellent. Here I go!* (Please excuse my spelling – I find myself shifting from Oxford, to Webster and back!) Remembering this helps me to recall when a group of community friends from Ontario got together to wish me bon voyage for my Ph.D. program. They presented me with a beautiful red-leather, gold-leaf Oxford dictionary! I was truly delighted with it and told them so – not saying a word about Webster in the USA! Oh – more to learn on my journey.

In my last year at U of T, I did field work with Mrs. Diane Allen in her district in Etobicoke, a western suburb of Toronto. Mrs. Allen was not only an excellent public health nurse but she also gave me many opportunities to serve on my own.

A thank you was given to me from D. B. McPherson, the Principal of Park Lawn School, which was where I worked with Mrs. Allen. The thank you was in the Park Lawn Home and School Association Bulletin, April, 1955.

What We Owe Each Child

A right to grow in body and mind,
A right to live in peace,
A right to hope, aspire, achieve
To study and knowledge increase.

A right to faith in God above,
A right to guidance wise,
A right to love, a right to truth,
All this we must enjoy.

The Church, home, school and community,
All are in one combined
To help our children a future to face,
With Courage and peace of mind.

May we always fulfill our duty well,
And never shrink from our task
The future generation depends on us,
Together – we must plan and act.

—Floris E. King, 1955

"We wish to thank Miss King, who wrote our series of articles entitled 'Viewing Health' which have appeared in our Bulletin. Miss King very modestly declined to be mentioned, but since we have had many inquiries about the articles, we felt that we should give her credit for such a fine piece of work. She is a graduate of the Toronto East General Hospital School of Nursing, who will have completed a three-year post-graduate course at the University of Toronto this spring for her Bachelor of Science in Nursing degree."

—D. B. McPherson, Park Lawn Home and School Bulletin, April, 1955

To conclude the school year, I wrote the Nursing School Hymn and presented it to Florence Emory, retiring Dean, School of Nursing, University of Toronto.

Our Hymn

Our Nursing School we cherish
Our laughs, our hopes, our fears;
New friendships, knowledge, faith untold,
Our strength for future years.

Our friendships all shall scatter,
Across the ocean wide,
But a part of us goes with them,
In heart and soul and mind.
We each shall live a better life,
For now we do belong,
To a heritage we are so proud,
U of T we will be strong.

And so with God's great mercy
May we always do our part,
To make this world a better place
For friendships everywhere.

—Floris E. King, 1955

The Etobicoke Health Department invited me to join them as a public health nurse. I joyously agreed.

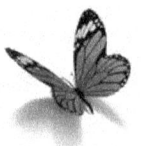

THREE

Public Health Nursing in Etobicoke, Ontario

1955 - 1958

After graduation, Dad took me to a car dealership (Chrysler) and we selected a car for me, a beautiful Plymouth. After passing the driving lessons and a written exam, we walked over for the car – and I drove us home. We were both so happy. All I had to promise was not to pick up someone on the side of the road.

So, here I was, driving to the Toronto suburb of Etobicoke to my first job, a public health nurse – in my new car. I must say, I had a big smile on my face!

The first week I was in the public health nurses' office. Ruth Kent was our Director of Nursing. A Gem! Orientation was a great week. I learned the details of my schedule and reviewed files. I learned about the various report formats and on what papers they were written. Mostly it was a get to know you time which included a lovely staff welcome party. By the end of the week I was eager to get going.

On Monday I went to one of my schools – Queen's Court School – grades kindergarten through sixth. The building looked new, but was actually a few years old.

I introduced myself to the principal, who went with me to my office and introduced me to the teachers along the way – very pleasant.

My office was large, bright and very well equipped. Our program was to care for cuts, bruises, and small accidents; to examine each child with an eye exam and take their weight; and prepare a family member (re: their questions, concerns, etc.) to be present when the doctor arrived for physicals for second and fifth graders. Also, a teacher could send a child to the nurse if the child appeared ill or upset. Each child brought in a physical report from his own doctor for kindergarten and grade 1 entrance. No child in the school required day medication.

So – there I was – going over the names of the children, setting up my records, and establishing a set of schedules.

My First Five Minutes at Queens Court School

And there I sat, poised, going over my list
When into my room, a wee 5 year old skipped.
Without a word, on tippie-toe stood,
Flicked on the light, and in he strode.
With door wide open, and in manly pose,
He carried on – accompanied by the trickling noise.

When he was all through, he fluttered the knob
Switched off the light – the end of the job!
He turned to me, and with a great wide grin,
Said "Hi" – and was off again.
I sat for a moment under the charm of his gaze,
And thought to myself: What a wonderful age!

My second school was a larger one – Queensway School – grades six to eight, in the middle of my district, Queensway. Monday, Wednesday, and Friday mornings I was at Queensway School; the responsibility of the Nurse was similar to Queens Court School. There I also taught a class called Baby

Sitting for Neighbors, designed a checklist to talk over with the parents, collected telephone numbers where the parents could be contacted, etc.

The Queensway School population was a reflection of the development in my Queensway District. During this time there was a large immigration of people from Italy, and I thought that most of the Italian families landed in my district!

The children at Queensway School were adorable – always a big smile, happy, well fed, and (what I noticed first) a beautiful, thick head of hair. When I arrived at the school, there was a line-up of children wanting to carry my bag in. At times I wished I had more bags!

The policy for the first year of the children admitted from Italy, who spoke and understood only Italian, was that they were admitted to the grade of their age group. The first year they were helped by both teachers and students. If, after Christmas, they were speaking some English (and most did), then they received assistance in writing English. There was no pressure put on them. Most were so eager and <u>very</u> happy, and some accomplished the reading and writing at their class level. Most of the children were in kindergarten or in the first grade. If any stress was observed by the teacher, I was brought into the discussion. The children responded well to a drink of water, holding hands, hugs, and sometimes lying down on our examination table and talking quietly. Sometimes their sobs were almost too much for the nurse! But comforting a little one helped us both. The teacher and I discussed at length how difficult it was for certain children when they would get upset or frustrated. We shared how best to prevent it or be aware of the child's behavior before it got to be too much for the student.

As there were older children who had gone through this adjustment period, I found them very helpful and encouraging with the little ones.

In making home visits, the older children, after coming home from school, would act as an interpreter for their parents and me. This would help the parents – so eager to do the very best for their children. If there was an illness, I would make an evening visit. Father, who was working, could help interpret for Mother and myself. I found my evening visits very helpful for us all.

Each afternoon I also did new baby visits. I soon picked up enough Italian for "bambino" visits. They'd know you as a P.H. nurse from your navy-blue dress or suit plus your bag. However, with my first few visits I had a problem. They required you to drink to the baby before undressing him/her (back then, babies were "mummied"). At the time, they made their own wine – in the kitchen. Very good but strong! After five baby visits in an afternoon and driving home… Well, I quickly learned it was the <u>process</u> of drinking to the baby, not <u>what</u> one drank. So I would make motions like I was driving, go to the water tap, fill a glass with water, and drink to the baby – all was well! Mama would give me a great wide grin.

Other responsibilities I had were home visits for other health problems, assistance and referrals. For example, the Lion's Club looked after children's glasses; Masonic Lodge looked after transportation for elderly regarding medical needs; Salvation Army would visit with the elderly in their homes, etc.

I also arranged with a local hospital so that I would come in and do new baby baths with the mother present. With mothers in hospital longer than they are now, this was possible. This also introduced me to new mothers in my district, so they would recognize me when I made a home visit later.

Besides all that, there were community responsibilities. I spoke as requested at the Lion's Club, etc., and at the Home and School Parents/Teachers monthly meetings – in both my schools.

One other responsibility I had which I thoroughly enjoyed was to be Chair of the Queensway Child Health Centre with four other PHNs and a doctor plus four Red Cross ladies to help check in the mothers, babies, and toddlers. They also provided apple juice, lemonade, etc. The CHC was conducted in the basement of the Anglican Church in my district. It was originally held once a month, but with arrival of the new Italian babies we had it three times a month. One session for Canadian mothers/babies and two for the Italian mothers/babies.

The babies were weighed (records kept) and the mother counseled by one of the five PHNs, as well as the doctor.

The Italian babies were beautiful, happy and very active. They were all breast fed. If mother ran out, she would pass her baby to a friend or someone else nearby to continue with the baby's feeding! Even though the children were healthy, I knew we were not meeting their needs. We automatically gave each mother a small bottle of cod liver oil and gestured to give one drop a day. On one of my home visits I was shocked to learn the cod liver oil drops were going in their ears, not mouth. All drops to them were eardrops!

I spoke to our Medical Officer of Health (MOH) – we had a problem! Despite all the visits, literature, and eardrops, we were not communicating. After learning we had one in Toronto, I asked if I could phone the Italian Consulate for interpreters. My MOH said I could if I thought it would help.

I did. I spoke with the consul and told him my concerns. It turned out he was a young man with a beautiful wife and a three-year-old child. He said, "I will send my wife out to your next Child Health Centre meeting and see what we can do."

What a lovely lady – wife of the Italian consul. She stayed, spoke with the women, held babies and arranged the following for us:

- eight interpreters for nurses, doctors and Red Cross teams;
- Italian newspapers to translate and print our literature into Italian – plus run off many copies too.

Soon the word got out that the Italian consul's wife was coming to our CHC. WOW! At our next clinic, mothers and babies were all dressed up and lined up around the church grounds. The doctor checked the ears of all the babies who had been given cod liver oil drops, all babies (and ears!) were alright.

The MOH spoke with me a couple of times and encouraged me to go on for a Master's of Public Health. He said he wanted to write a letter of reference when I decided where I was going. And he did – a very honourable MOH.

I decided on the University of Michigan, School of Public Health, in Ann Arbor, Michigan.

An Aside

Thirty years ago I received a Christmas note from the manager of the Red Cross Volunteers at the CHC in Queensway District, Etobicoke, Ontario. She said she wanted me to know that the numbers I cut out from the calendar and covered with scotch tape are still used. The numbers were used to keep the order of those who arrived. Some of the numbers were missing, but she said they know which ones and still use the ones that are left. What beautiful people. OH MY – I missed them.

I paused quietly for at least half an hour. How lovely! What a beautiful person she is, to have written a note to me. I wrote her immediately and expressed my thanks and love. What a great setting! Some settings and people can be so evil and damaging, but not at Queensway District, Etobicoke, Ontario, Canada.

FOUR

University of Michigan School of Public Health, Ann Arbor, Michigan, USA

1958 - 1959

I moved into a new graduate residence, Markley Hall, with Mrs. Atwood as our house mother. It was a beautiful residence, and just a few steps from the School of Public Health.

The University program was excellent. I took courses in statistics, epidemiology, education, health education and sociology. I also planned and organized a Christmas Concert. I drove to Raleigh (after receiving permission from the Dean) and rented a piano for the auditorium. A student choir and I met weekly to prepare our program. I wanted some children too, so the Dean's wife organized a car pool for Saturday mornings. We had a great time practicing.

When we performed, the concert hall was completely full – including the steps which were covered with babies in bassinettes! It was a great Christmas celebration.

Dolores Belongia, from Wisconsin, was my roommate. Dolores was in a different program from me; she was at the School of Nursing. We enjoyed each other and laughed and laughed! I visited Dolores's home in Wisconsin, and Dolores came to mine in Toronto in July. With coming "north" to Canada, her mother made sure she came warmly dressed! Flannelette pajamas, sweaters, etc. Her first comment as we were driving from the airport to my home was, "Oh, you have paved roads!" Well, after she got initiated with drives to Niagara Falls and many parts of Ontario and Quebec. We laughed and laughed about the winter gear!

The year went quickly by. I became particularly fond of epidemiology and statistics. I did well in my studies and was elected into the Delta Omega Honor Society. My mother was invited to visit the program – I'm not so sure she knew what was happening, other than it was good. Mabel Rugan, my professor, explained it to her.

There were several groups who came to the campus, asking that I consider working with their program. I selected the Ontario TB Association/Thoracic Society as well as the Ontario Department of Health. There was a need to study the 47 Counties in Ontario regarding their health needs, concerns and resources. I happily accepted the challenge. My title was Director of Health Education for the Province of Ontario.

At the time, I recalled a verse by Ralph Waldo Emerson:

"What lies behind us
And what lies before us
Are tiny matters compared
To what lies within us."

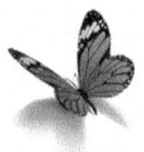

FIVE

Study of Health Needs, Concerns, and Resources of 47 Counties of Ontario, Canada, Health Education Director, Ontario TB Association and within the Province of Ontario

1959 - 1964

*L*ooking at the map of Ontario, there were 47 Counties. Each one had an MHO (Medical Health Officer), public health department with PHNs (Public Health Nurses), small defined communities with churches, schools and local hospitals. That was my base.

I went to Eddie S. O'Brien, Director of the Ontario TB and Thoracic Society, with the proposal to visit each of the 47 counties for a week – which, with writing the report, would take me a year. The report would analyze findings and make specific recommendations. I would stay in a hotel or motel for Sunday through Thursday and drive home Friday to Toronto. When accommodation in a hotel or motel was not available, I would stay with a family. All this was approved by E.S. O'Brien and the Board of Directors of the Ontario TB Association.

Each week was a full week's effort! I returned to Toronto each weekend to catch my breath and give my reports to Norma Lytle, our secretary at the office. She was such a great person.

My goal was to do a preliminary assessment of health problems, concerns, and needs as identified by the MOH, PHNs, principals and select teachers who expressed interest in supporting and helping, as well as church groups, police, judges, and presidents of local organizations and clubs. To book these initial visits, I telephoned these "Community Ladies and Gentlemen" and invited them to a meeting for the purpose of reviewing in some detail what our goals were: to know and understand the health needs of their communities as well as provide a structure which would address these needs/concerns.

So we identified the problems and concerns of each county in the province of Ontario. One of their aspirations was to establish a health council and chairperson voted in by the community leaders. In this way, the provinces of Ontario and the Ontario TB Association would help with the health needs and concerns as identified. Plus, the Ontario TB Association was planning, with the University of Toronto, to have a yearly one-week workshop for the chairs of each of the councils in Ontario. The purpose of the workshops was to develop knowledge and skills and share accomplishments. The workshops would be held in the summer so that student residents would be available. This proved a great success, and at the first workshop at the University, each participant received a certificate with their name on it!

I again was encouraged to go on with my education, to get a Ph.D. I decided, after tours around and interviews, that the University of North Carolina at Chapel Hill, North Carolina, was for me. I was delighted to learn that the Board of Directors of the Ontario TB Association offered me a scholarship to complete my Ph.D. – they didn't want to lose me!

A few years later, I learned that the 47 Councils had been combined into only 5 Councils. Sounds great to me – you are great!

A complete report was done of the year's work which was used as a basis for development of resources by the Provincial Health Department, Provincial Education Department, Roads Department, and of course, the Health Department.

The joy of meeting all these community leaders and working through their concerns was a remarkable experience.

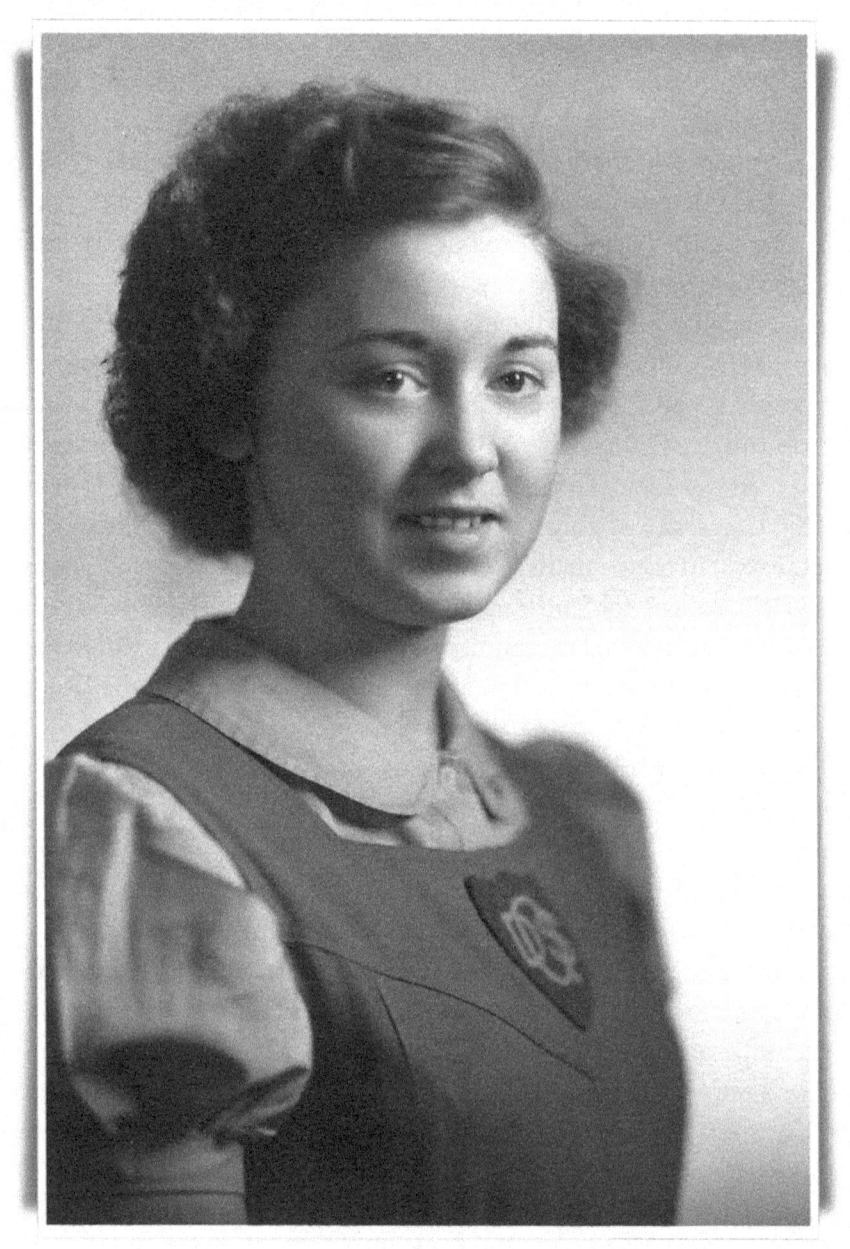

Floris E. King
Qu' Appelle Diocesan Girls School,
Regina, Saskatchewan, 1941

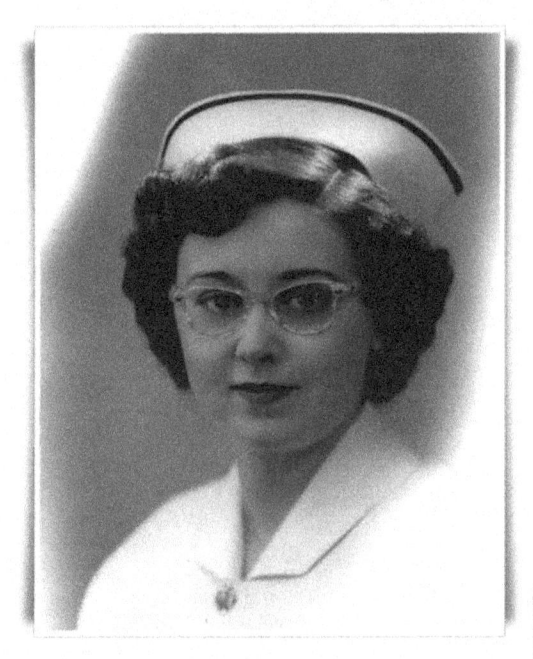

Floris E. King, T.E.G.H., 1951
Registered Nurse
Toronto East General Hospital,
Toronto, Ontario

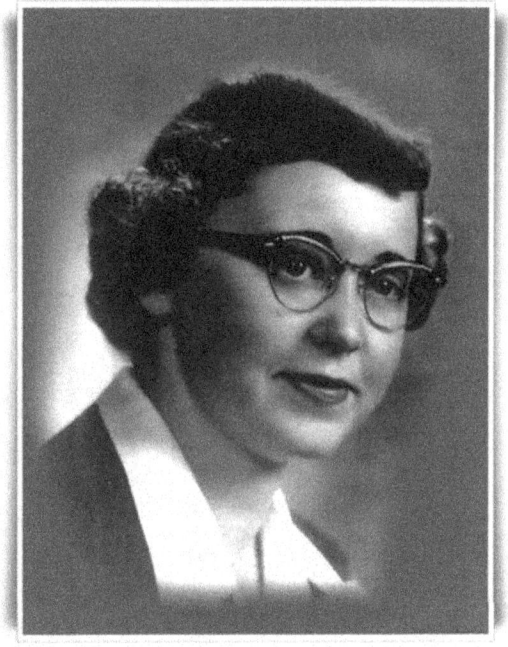

Floris E. King, Ph.D.
University of North Carolina, 1967,
School of Public Health
Chapel Hill, North Carolina

SCHOLARLY PURSUIT OF NURSING SCIENCE

> To Floris
>
> You are Canada's Number One Nurse today ~
> And your colleagues are rightfully proud
> Of your record of worthy accomplishments
> That single you out from the crowd.
>
> You're our School's foremost academician
> And our leader (where leadership counts!)
> You have dignity, poise, integrity and
> Compassion in generous amounts!
>
> Thus we offer our congratulations ~
> But there's more ~ so much more ~
> we would say;
> You're our King of Research
> but our
> Queen of Heart ~
> And our hearts are all with you today!
>
> From your many friends on UBC's nursing faculty

University of British Columbia, 1971
UBC faculty recognition, plus silver candlesticks.
Presented to me at a dinner held for me by the faculty, following the first Canadian Nursing Research Conference in Ottawa.

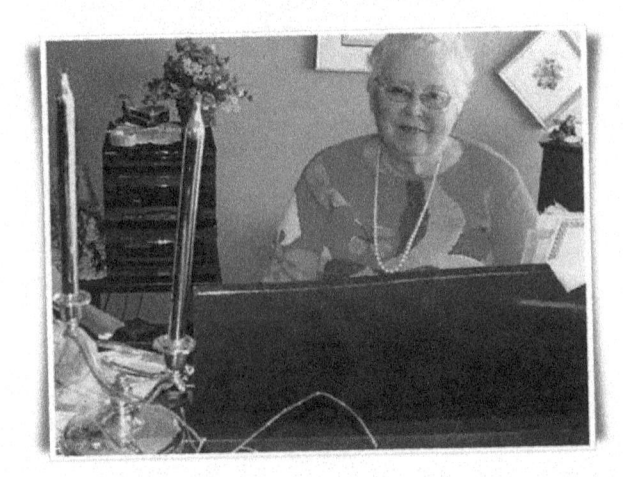

UBC facility, 2008.

Please note the silver candlestick holder you presented to me at a dinner upon my return from Ottawa — Canada's first national research conference, held in 1971. It has traveled with me every place I've moved to since. Thank you.

SCHOLARLY PURSUIT OF NURSING SCIENCE 23

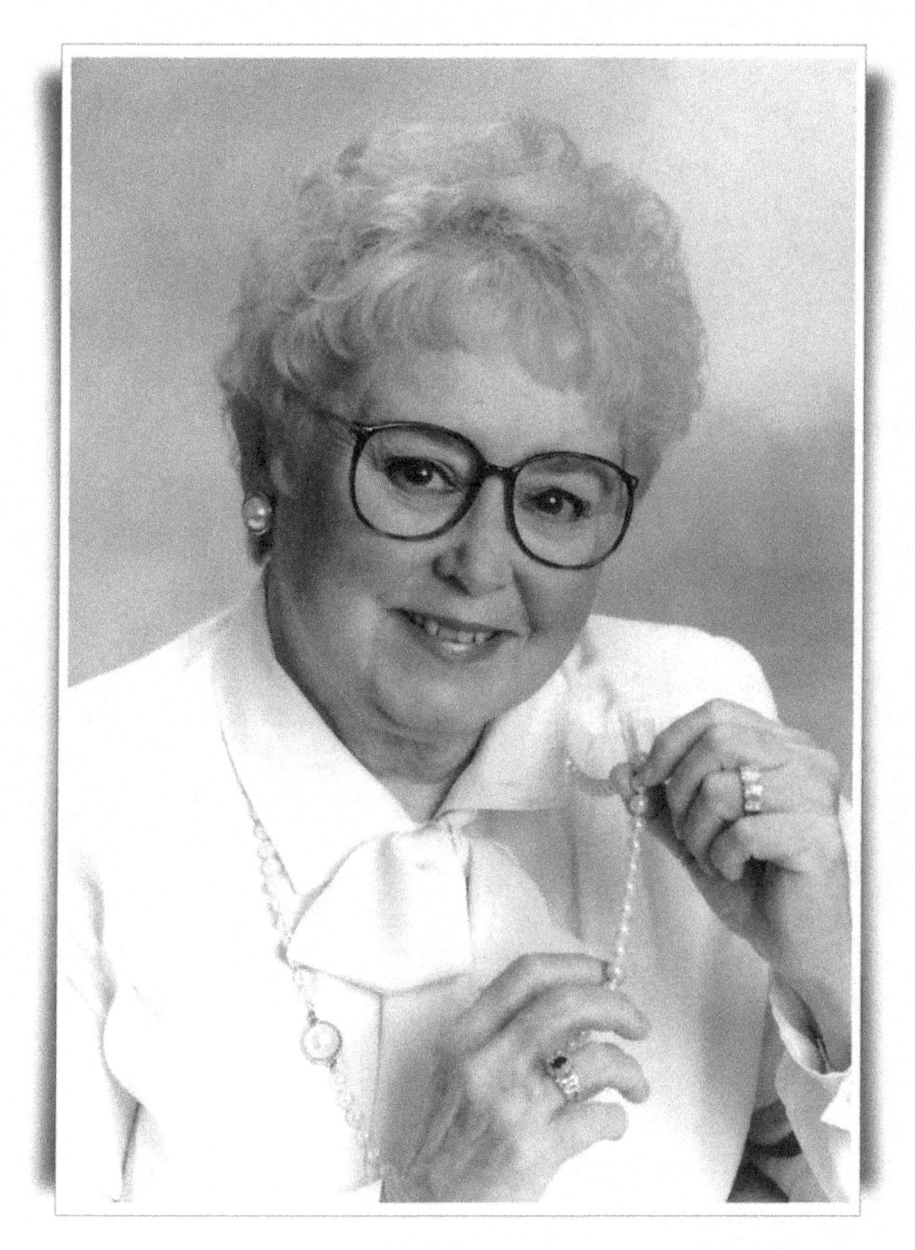

Lady Floris E. King Ph.D.
Retired 1992
University of Minnesota School of Nursing
Professor Emeritus

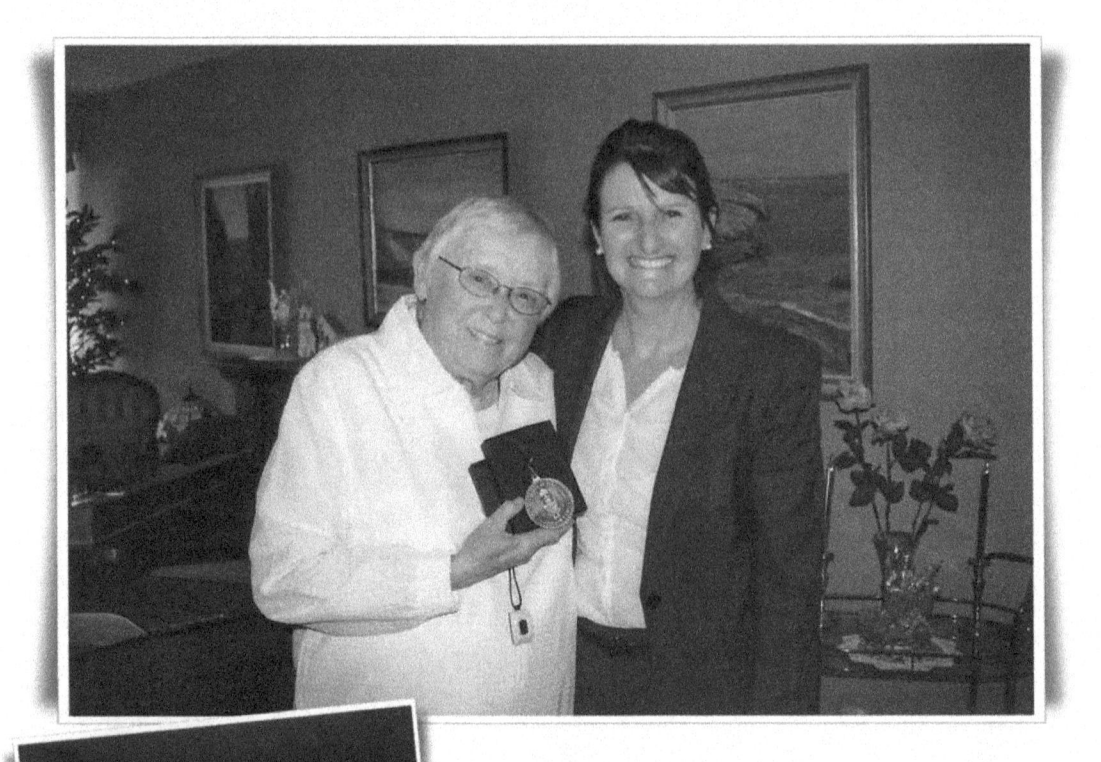

24 SCHOLARLY PURSUIT OF NURSING SCIENCE

Dean Nelson, School of Nursing, University of Toronto.

She flew to me in Minneapolis to present an award of Top Graduate of the School of Nursing–Peer Voted–celebrating the 90th year of the Faculty of Nursing, University of Toronto, August 22, 2011. I was so appreciative.

Unfortunately, I was not well enough to travel to Toronto.

Lin and Lu, PHNs Taiwan (Directors), 1985

They spent spring quarter with me then returned home after completing their research study to finish the design (in Chinese) at home.

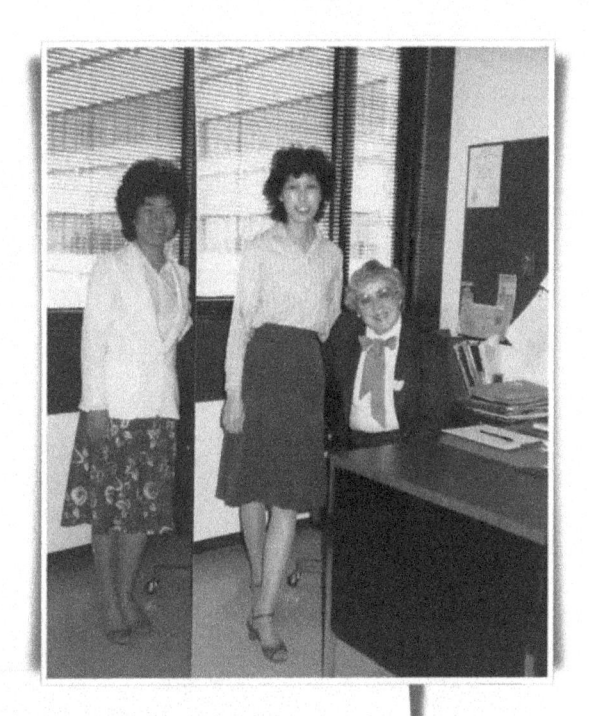

You're always up to something...

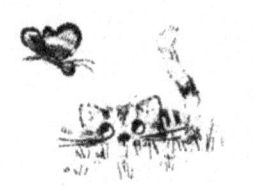

Dear Dr. King:

...and it's always something nice!

Thanks So Much!

Ming-Haou Lu and Gong-Yu Lin

Professor Sirrka Lauri and me, in my University of Minnesota office, discussing my visit to University of Kuopio, Finland.

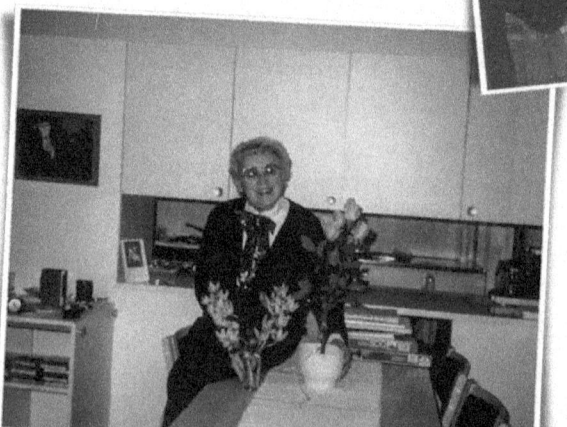

University of Kuopio apartment for guest professors (at University of Kuopio).

Pirrko Mikkanen: With your English and spirit, you made my life full of joy—thank you, thank you, thank you—Dr. Floris King (you are so brilliant).

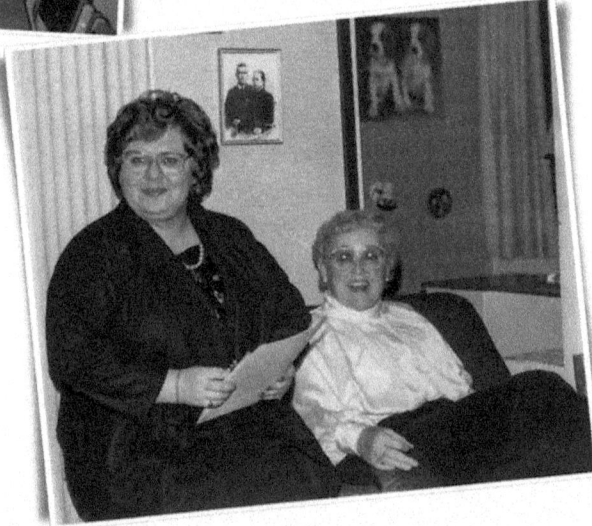

SCHOLARLY PURSUIT OF NURSING SCIENCE   27

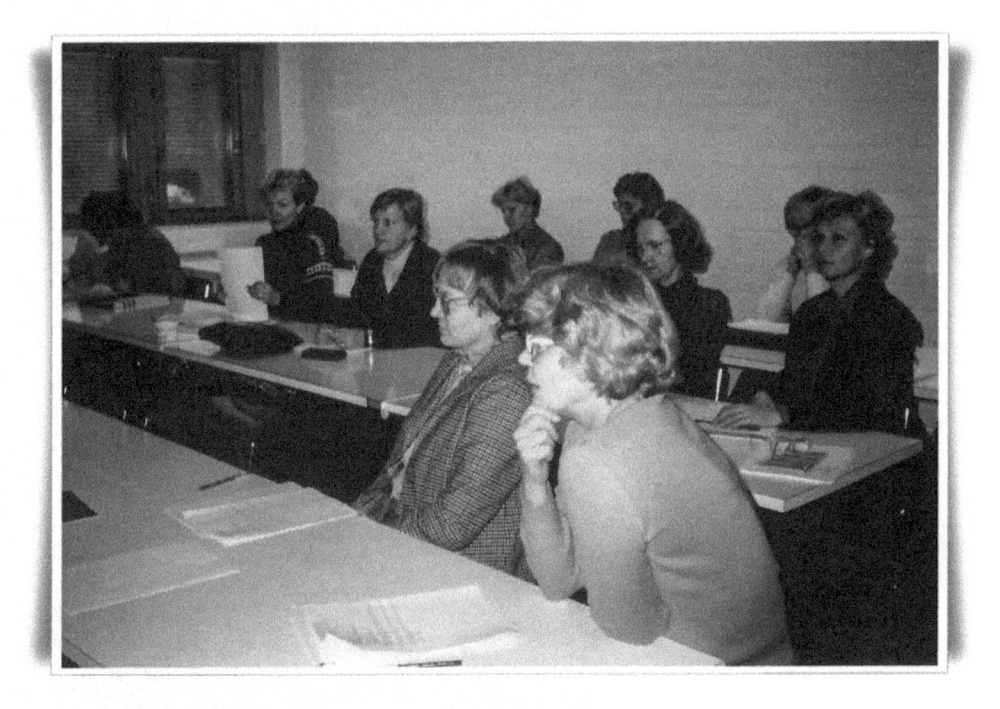

Some of our doctoral students I taught, University of Kuopio. Many traveled overnight by train.

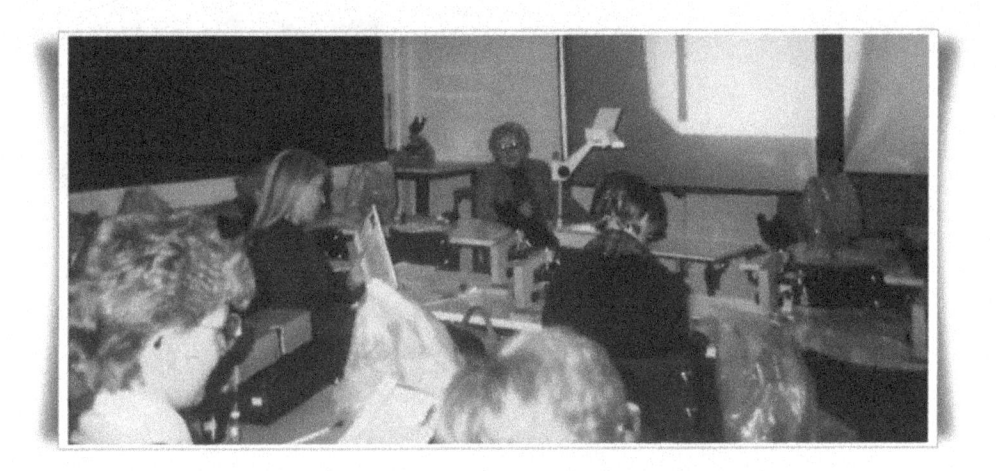

Some of the master's students I taught, University of Kuopio.

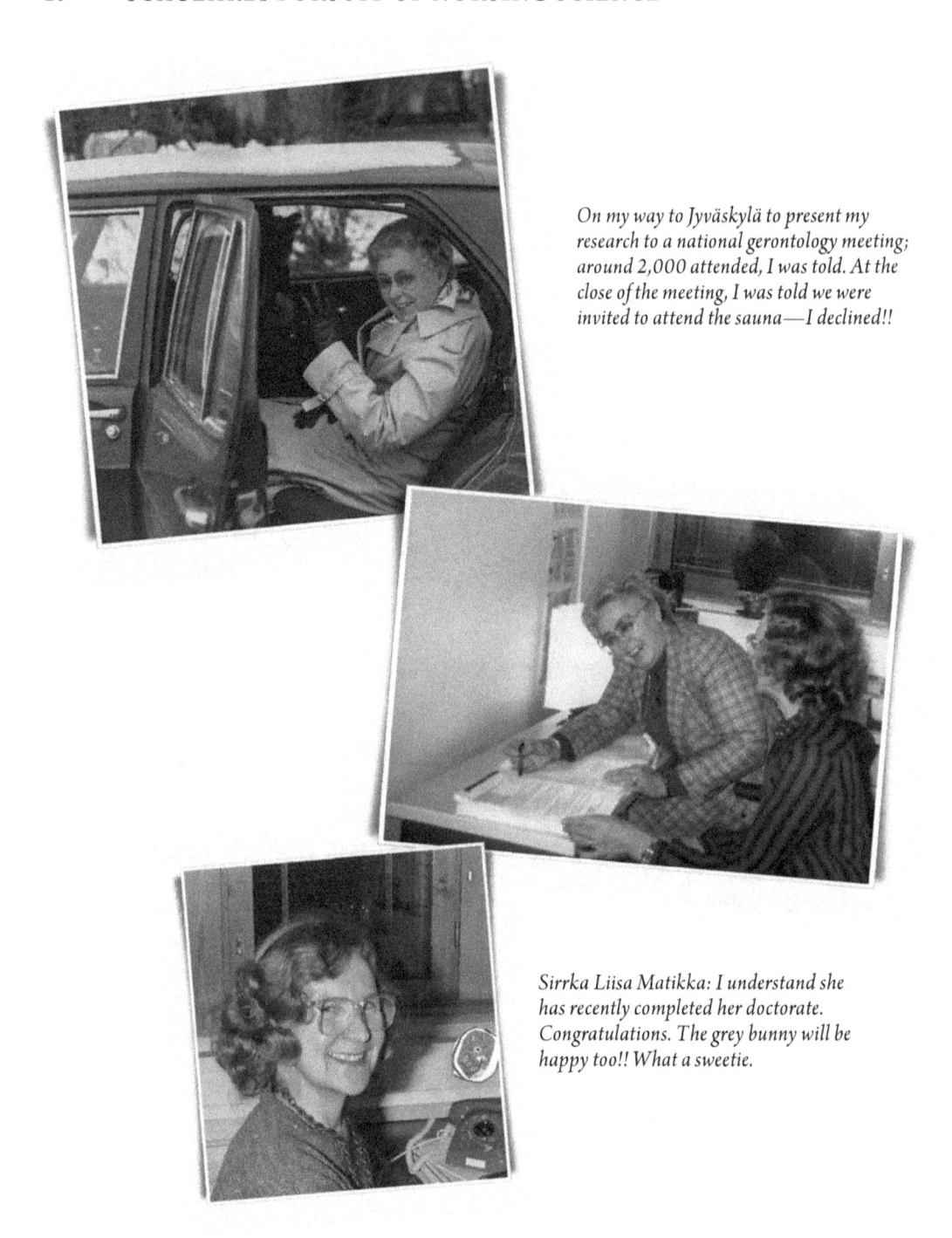

On my way to Jyväskylä to present my research to a national gerontology meeting; around 2,000 attended, I was told. At the close of the meeting, I was told we were invited to attend the sauna—I declined!!

Sirrka Liisa Matikka: I understand she has recently completed her doctorate. Congratulations. The grey bunny will be happy too!! What a sweetie.

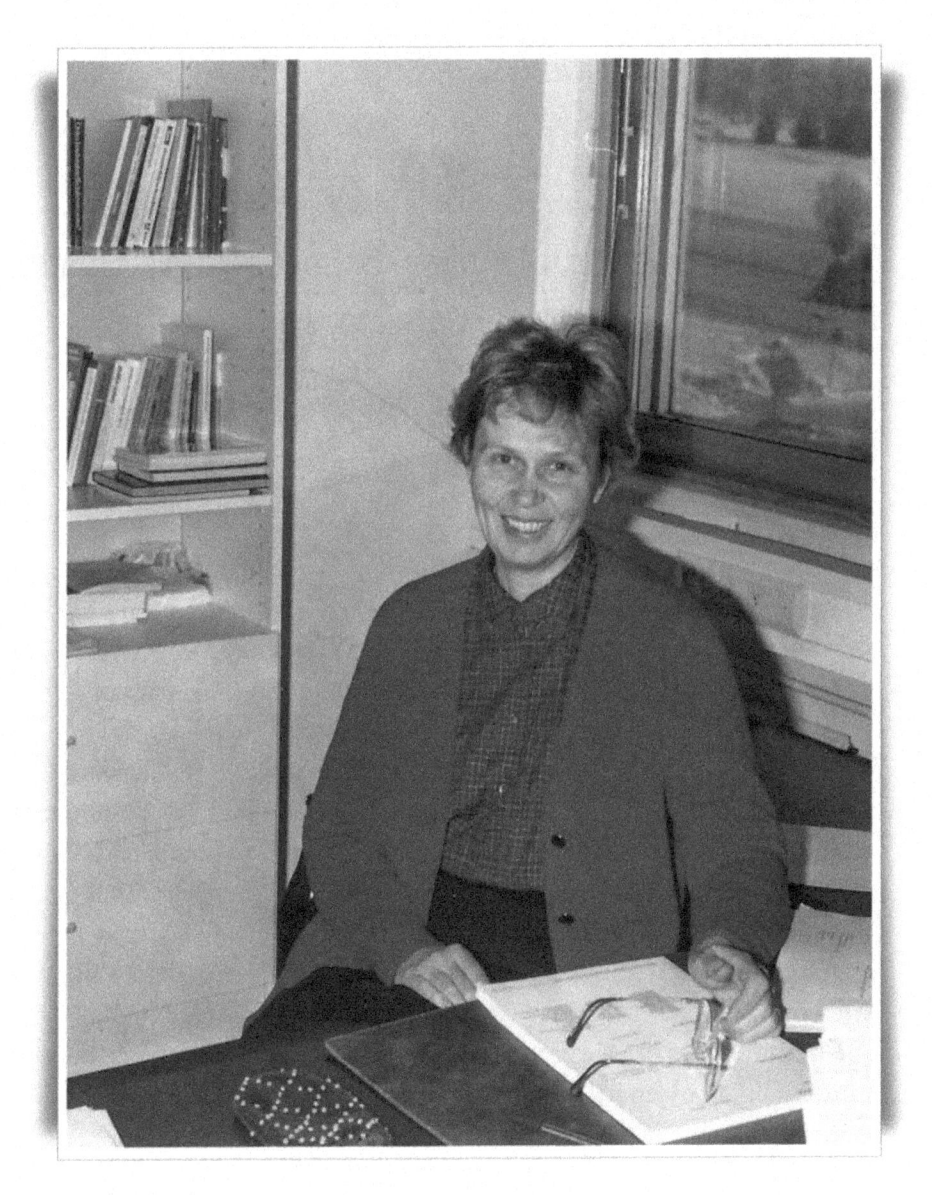

Professor Sirrka Lauri: A brilliant, capable nurse whom I've been proud to meet. Happy Retirement! You are special and an outstanding daughter violinist.

SIX

University of North Carolina, School of Public Health, Chapel Hill, North Carolina, Ph.D. Program

1964 -1967

My advisor at Chapel Hill was Lucy Morgan, a knowledgeable and lovely lady. My program was selected by the two of us as was my dissertation. When Lucy retired, Ralph Boatman became my advisor. As this was my last fling as a full-time student, I tried to pursue as much varied education as I could! I took sociology, epidemiology, and statistics - a bit of a handful with also having to learn German. French I passed, of course, the first time around. But that German! It took me two attempts to get a pass. Two languages were required to obtain a Ph.D. at that time and German was a requirement of the Ph.D. program.

Poetry is my joy, and German poetry is so beautiful. I could never have learned German without poems. I was put in a German class along with students who had had four years of high school German. I had never even sneezed in German! Geshundheit – to your health! However, the second time trying, I passed it!

Gedenkvers

Weist du, was Leben sei?
ein ewig Wiederfinden
Drum, wie die Jahre schwinden,
sprich nie das Wort: vorbei.

—Rudolf Alexander Schröder

Remember

Do you know what life is?
An eternal finding again
Therefore, as the year ends
Speak not the word: gone.

My Father died. Multiple strokes. I flew home. I watched the moon all the way. I tried to plan all that would be required – meeting family that was flying in, selecting a casket (at the time I didn't know that the cost of the casket was the cost of the funeral), etc. I learned fast. All the family went down the aisle two by two – not one noticed that I was alone. But then I realized DAD was with me all the way as he always had been.

This poem I wrote, hoping someday I will be with him again – soon.

My Father – Following a Song – With Me

If I die
Before I wake
As the little prayer says
Please God, take.

Be not sad
Nor either forlorn
For unless I'm wrong
I'm following a song.

Now I walk
In forest green
Where pain is not present
Nor felt, seen.

But birds, butterflies are there
With orchestral music everywhere
Where there is love and joy
For all to share - AMEN

—Floris E. King, 1966

"A DIFFERENT WORLD CANNOT BE BUILT
BY INDIFFERENT PEOPLE."

—Dad's favourite saying

SEVEN

Director of Programs, Nursing, Nursing Consultant, National TB and Thoracic Society, Ottawa, Canada

1967 - 1968

I went on to work in Ottawa, Canada, living in Elfin Apartments on the top floor within a block of our office. Dr. C. W. L. Jeans was our director and excellent, indeed. Anne Grant, with an "e," Bettie Sutherland (both sweethearts) and myself were on staff, along with the Christmas Seal Director.

I reviewed my dissertation: "Historical Study of the Voluntary Community Health Program in Canada with Projective Emphasis." I planned a summary review for each province – this for the purpose of triggering further thoughts, ideas and suggestions from each province.

I also prepared an overall synthesis for all of Canada. This was supported by the five specific charts comparing year by year progress in community activities, which was also in the dissertation.

Once I reviewed all this with the National TB and Thoracic Society of Ontario and Canada, I received their comments and recommendations on utilizing my dissertation for future planning.

My secretary and I prepared all the materials for each province, and I proceeded to visit with each of them. It was so good to see them again, but the TV stations followed me too much! At each place I visited, the TV stations put me on for interviews. This was also helpful for each provincial organization to get the publicity.

The discussion was remarkable with many thoughts and ideas for the future. I was both surprised and delighted. At first I wondered if an historical review would or could be so helpful in looking to the future. It was.

I learned much from writing the dissertation as well as presenting it.

By this time, I was receiving several requests to join a faculty position in a University. Dr. Jeans said he knew he would not be able to keep me for long, but that I had been most helpful, and we all had a "filling" dinner together. I was so happy and so very thankful. I needed to help other settings so much. I was uncertain in what direction I would go – but I knew I must try.

EIGHT

University of British Columbia, Department of Nursing, Associate Professor, Director to Launch New Masters Program in Nursing, Vancouver

1968 - 1971

I had excellent experience as a student at Universities. I eagerly drove to Vancouver hoping much was to be learned as a faculty person. It was good to add that hesitant thought, as I later learned.

I was asked to become the Director of the new Masters in Nursing Program with a focus on continuity of care of the elderly at home. I was delighted. Many Canadians retire in Vancouver and the outlying areas of British Columbia, much as Florida is a retirement place for elderly Americans. My parents and I (as a child) came to Vancouver every summer. It was like a return home; there were not too many changes.

As I was coming at the end of August with the admissions of the first class (a two-year program) starting the first week of September, I asked several questions prior to coming:

1. Has the program been approved by the Graduate Committee of the School? *Response: Yes*
2. Have the courses been approved by the Nursing School Graduate Committee? *Response: Yes*

3. Have the courses been approved by the Graduate School? *Response: Yes*
4. Has the M. Sc. N. been approved by the Graduate School? *Response: Yes*
5. Have Departments on Campus, which will be having our graduate students, approved having them? *Response: Yes*

Upon arriving at the end of August, I found the questions had been incorrectly answered – all except #2 should have been answered "No"! I was startled! I worked day and night.

Our final approval, plus course work, came through in spring, with the Graduate School and the other scholarly departments approving almost immediately. The Department of Statistics refused having the nurses, as they thought they could not learn statistics! Well, I decided that I would take my nights and write a Statistical Manual for Nursing – just keeping ahead of the students. In Canada, courses are a year long with six to eight subjects taken at a time. The year gives students time to do many in-depth papers, increasing understanding of the subject. Tests were usually held every three to four months depending on the subject. With statistics, I tested the students every two weeks. I asked each student to not only keep their class notes but also a book on their biweekly test results. With the students' permission, I took these results to the Statistics Department at the end of the year.

The Department of Statistics opened their doors to nursing students the next year.

My days were full with working with the Graduate Faculty. Preparation of several courses had been started but not all. Mostly, I made sure the students' schedules were understood and advisors for each student were set up.

The second year at UBC I submitted a proposal to the Federal Government of Canada for funding: "Canada's First National Nursing Research Conference." To my surprise and joy it got funded with the request that the Conference be held in Ottawa and be conducted in English and French. I agreed. I asked our Alumni Association for HELP! They were so wonderful and supportive and helpful too! I loved them!

You must remember UBC's Master's Program was only the second in Canada. Research was relatively new for Nursing in Canada.

The UBC Alumni Organization had 60 (the number registered for the conference from across Canada) leather daffodils corsages made for each of us to wear, and boxes and boxes of yellow daffodils were shipped from Vancouver to Ottawa. The weather in Vancouver, in February, is beautiful – whereas Ottawa is still in the dead of winter. The members of the Alumni Association also spent evenings with us to help us keep up with the mailings. They were wonderful! I especially respected their kindness and support.

The Canadian Nurses Association is located in Ottawa. They too were readily available for the Conference to help with the many tasks that there always were. What a delight to get nursing research at the national front.

When I got home to Vancouver all the faculty had a dinner for me and presented me with a silver two-candlestick holder engraved: "First Canadian Nursing Research Conference 1971." It still sits on my grand piano, and I enjoy it with a warm smile. They also wrote me a poem! They knew I loved poems – in our first year together I tended to keep us all going with little poems!

"To Floris

You are Canada's Number
One Nurse today –
And your Colleagues are
Rightfully proud
Of your record of worthy
Accomplishments
That single you out from
The crowd.

> *You're our School's fore-*
> *Most academician*
> *And our leader (where*
> *Leadership counts!)*
> *You have dignity, poise*
> *Integrity and*
> *Compassion in generous amounts!*
>
> *Thus we offer our*
> *Congratulations*
> *But there's more –*
> *We would say:*
> *You're our <u>King</u> of Research –*
> *But our*
> *Queen of Heart*
> *And our hearts are all*
> *With you today."*
>
> —1971

(I wept for joy then; I weep for their love today).

In early 1971 a new Director of the School arrived – Muriel Uprichard, with a Ph.D. in psychology from a University somewhere in California. I helped her find a house to rent near the school, with a good fenced yard for her dog. I drove her about to find different things for her home (when you are new, it is difficult to know where to go to find things).

Within a week of School starting, Dr. Uprichard asked me down to her office. She immediately said, "I am going to be the only Ph.D. person in this School, and I am telling you early, so you can prepare to get out. You have a tenure vote coming up, and I will see that you do not get the votes…"

I was thunderstruck. My legs were so wobbly I could scarcely make it back to my office. I thought, "Those faculty know what I have done here – we got along very well – they will never vote against me." But the day came, and Dr. Uprichard had indicated that to be in her favor they had to vote against me, as she was going to be the only Ph.D. in the School. There were those who voted YES, but one too many voted NO. So this is the justice of University life – my first experience with faculty politics.

I could hardly get to my apartment; I was completely numb. Two of my colleagues, Rosie Murakami and Pauline Capelle, supported me for the next few weeks. I had received several letters after the research conference, requesting I consider an appointment with them (what to do?). I left with great sadness.

NINE

Dalhousie University, School of Nursing
Halifax, Nova Scotia, Canada

1971 – 1974

I flew to Halifax from Vancouver for my interview with Dean MacDonald, under whom the School of Nursing was structured.

I was assured that the Administration of the School would receive every consideration and support. The previous director had been there 20 years and was beloved.

With my visit I noted several items for discussion:

- There was no meeting with faculty as my examination time was taking place;
- Administrative structure – School of Nursing was under the Dean of Pharmacy;
- Physical structure of Nursing program was scattered into several buildings – an old house was used for administration. It was indicated that plans were underway for a new School of Nursing Building.
- Financial support for a new faculty with doctoral preparation was discussed – I was assured this too was being considered.

- The need to develop a Master's (regional) program with four maritime provinces; the need to explore and discuss needs, resources, and financial support.

The President and the Dean both indicated their support with the assurance they would work with me on behalf of the faculty of nursing.

My individual interviews with the present faculty revealed uncertainty and discomfort because they had enough workload, they said, and did not wish to conduct research and write it up. "Here in the Maritimes, we don't need it." They informed me that they were happy with the previous Dean, who had been with them for many years.

I still felt the challenges of new development could be made more stimulating. Two of my previous faculty from Vancouver followed me to Halifax. They were excellent leaders. But likewise, they were not well received. Faculty seemed determined – no more "extra work."

At each faculty meeting, I shared how we were doing so far, and always the question of workload came up. I had reviewed this question with them individually, but there was a growing NO.

So that's the way we started, with the focus on faculty growth, program development, and council work.

The Planning Council

From each province (New Brunswick, Prince Edward Island, Newfoundland and Labrador, and Nova Scotia) there were representatives from Nurses in Public Health, Nurses in Hospitals, Nurse-Midwives, Medical and Nursing Associations, plus Faculty of Dalhousie School of Nursing representatives.

We met once a month initially at the Nova Scotia Nurses' Association Meeting Room. There was much eagerness displayed for a nurses' master's program.

Our faculty meetings brought faculty up to date as well as answered questions and received comments.

I sensed some improvement in attitudes and offered more discussions. No requests were received, but I continued with our usual meetings. Dean MacDonald, our Dean was away for a couple of months, but I knew he wanted me to carry on.

One day, my secretary said she didn't know if I knew the faculty was meeting with the President in the afternoon. I said that I hadn't had a notice from the president or from any member of the faculty.

At this time, I learned that a member of the Dean's Council (of which I was also a member) had been meeting privately and individually with each of my faculty regarding their dissatisfaction with me. This person never spoke with me about what he was doing – well, I was shocked.

I phoned the president's office (as Dean MacDonald was still away) and asked for a morning appointment with him. I was stunned by what I learned from him.

The President said the faculty was dissatisfied with me. I asked why I hadn't been a part of this meeting. He said they asked to speak with him. I said how distressed I was with this situation, and asked that we both speak with the faculty along with the Council member who spoke with each of my faculty about me. Before Dean MacDonald had left, he had mentioned how satisfied he was with the development of the Council, including representatives from the Maritimes. He commented that this model would be used in developing future graduate courses.

There was nothing I could do or suggest that was acceptable, and there was no answer as to why this faculty member undertook this mission that seemed to me as underhanded. With tears in my eyes, I resigned. The President said my salary would continue until I was resettled elsewhere. Devastated, I went and picked up my things then went to a desolate park and just stayed in my car for hours.

In the meantime, over the previous two months, I had been receiving at least two telephone calls a week from Dean Irene Ramey at Texas Woman's University to come and work with her. I asked her why.

Dean Ramey said that at the time she was at Texas Woman's University (which I knew) but was moving to the University of Minnesota. The University of Minnesota needed leadership to develop a Ph.D. in Nursing Program. And since she'd seen my CV – she knew I could do it. In the year at Denton I could experience the doctoral program there, get my social security number and she would sign the yearly "science visa" until I got my green card while in Minnesota. She wanted me to come to the University of Minnesota as associate dean, with tenure and become the Director of the Ph.D. Program when the grant got approved.

Although I was too shattered to continue with anything with the name of any University attached to it, I thought it was not my nature to give up. So I did say yes to Dean Ramey. The thought of having the privilege to develop a doctoral program was what gave me a push.

TEN

Texas Woman's University, Denton, Texas, USA.

Professor, Associate Dean, and Director of Ph.D. in Nursing Program

1974 – 1975

Texas – boy was it hot – and I had thought it was mighty hot at UNC, North Carolina! But there were more snakes there – oh dear – and another move.

I arrived on a Monday morning in September. Dr. Kathryn Burnett was the Dean. Dean Burnett told me I had two doctoral courses to teach next day – an immediate start.

- N. 6553 Formulation and Testing of Hypothesis in Nursing
- N. 6560 Nursing Research Practicum

What a lovely group of students. Soon I met with the Doctoral Council. What an absolute delight. Dr. Peggy Chin and Dr. Elaine Mansfield were two of the members I specifically recall, but all of us had a great time working together. I couldn't believe the joy of being together with such research-oriented faculty.

I was taken to a building downtown to sign up for my social security number. It was a great moment – I was legal. The next challenge was the State Board of Nurses of Texas. They refused to accept my nurse licensure from Ontario, Canada, 1951. I appealed six times – still NO.

Knowing I was going to Minneapolis, I also requested acceptance of my Ontario licensure from the Minnesota State Board of Nursing – NO! So I borrowed many books and studied. July 13, 14, 15, 1975, I wrote the State Board exams in Austin, Texas – all alone again – and did great!

It was a great year – excellent students, wonderful scholars. I learned MUCH about doctoral programs, AND I became a legal immigrant with a science visa and a state licensure. WOW! Then it was another move, this time to Minneapolis. I felt a bit like a NOMAD! But I was determined to do my best.

ELEVEN

University of Minnesota, School of Nursing, Minneapolis, Minnesota, USA, Professor, Associate Dean, Director of Graduate Program, Doctoral Program Proposal Grant Writer, and Director of Approval of Ph.D. in Nursing Program

Two Nurse Scholars, Lin and Lu, Spend a Research Quarter and Return with a Research Proposal in 1983

1975 – 1991

The drive up to Minnesota from Denton was a mighty long one. I stored my furniture in Minneapolis and took off for the shore of Black Point (a cottage), Nova Scotia for the summer. My friend Jean Church and I walked the shore every day, climbed huge rocks, attended all summer celebrations at the shore's small towns – many lobster fests, children's carriage and doll parades, bag pipe parades. We went to many neighbor parties, read many books and did whatever the spirit moved us to do. It was a renewing summer.

I returned to Minneapolis in August, 1975, purchased my condo, had the condo redecorated completely and my furniture retrieved. I drove to the University School of Nursing but didn't go in. The last week of August, I went in to find where I would be working.

The Associate Dean responsibilities were waiting for me, as were the chair of the Graduate Counsel and the need to get the doctoral grant written. I visited parts of the nursing community to learn their expectations and needs for a doctoral program. Plus I volunteered for the Graduate School of Research Review Committee (for University Reviews) to learn about their review process and also to let them get to know me and my work.

In writing the Doctoral Grant I first established the Doctoral Committee – Dean Ramey made recommendations. It would have been more helpful to know that a grant had been submitted a year previously by two people, whom she recommended, and was not funded. It was one year later in reviewing some files that I found this out – might have helped me knowing this. However, we worked through our being together and the Grant was submitted. We received approval of the grant proposal - $438,000!

During this time two lovely Taiwanese public health nurse scholars arrived to spend a quarter to study nursing research with me and to write a research proposal to take home to administer.

Barbara O'Grady and her staff, plus other PHN's, met with the nurse specialists at my home. Lin and Lu were very special scholars and a delight to have visit.

Then I received word from Immigration that I could pick up my green card – what a relief! I just had one more step to become an American citizen – I would do it.

The only problem was that I had to return to my port of exit (Halifax) in order to pick it up. I asked Dean Ramey for a couple of days to do that. The answer was NO! So I arranged to fly Friday night, pick up my green card Saturday, and fly back Sunday. I sat on my carpet in the middle of my living room, holding my card, and wept buckets – I did it! I made up my mind I was immediately going for my citizenship, as I loved the USA and I insisted on being able to vote!

I went through all the process, but I was called back twice for my fingerprints, which I didn't understand at all. Soon, an FBI letter arrived with an appointment for me to see an FBI agent. Oh, all those steps leading up to the FBI Building in St. Paul – I was so frightened, but I was determined to make that appointment.

I found the door, knocked, and a deep voice said to come in. This big man was standing behind his desk. He looked at me and said, "You have no fingerprints."

I looked at my fingers and said, "Really? Perhaps it is because I have been playing the piano since I was three years old."

"Oh – that's it!" he boomed. "We have the same trouble with Arturo Toscanini." He then motioned me out. With a great wide grin on my face, I thought, boy, I was in good company and skipped down all those stairs and went home.

It wasn't long before I was a USA citizen. Inez Hinsvark had a cake covered with flags at home waiting for me. Nearly all of the public health nurses and Barbara O'Grady filled the courtroom. Inez was the only School of Nursing person present.

What a great day. I was given a small flag, and it is still attached to the top of my bed.

Then Dean Fahy arrived as our new Dean. At our first Doctoral Committee meeting, she came and said she wanted to rewrite the proposal in her style, and the proposal would go forward in her name. The Committee was astounded, and we said NO – we had already rewritten six of the proposals. But by our next meeting, I was not included. The Doctoral proposal went forward under Dean Fahy's name with the others' approval, I guess – no one would speak to me about this. I was devastated and completely ignored because I did not agree with Dean Fahy taking over my grant.

At this time, a young lady, Sirkka Sinkkonen (Lauri) was visiting from Finland. She said she heard about my Research course and asked if I would come to the University of Kuopio to teach and do research. I knew not a word of Finnish. She had arranged for a Fulbright Scholarship. I said yes and went, as exhausted as I was. I made all the arrangements and invited Jean Church to go with me. Jean retired early after the happenings at Dalhousie University.

Jean and I met in New York, and off we went.

TWELVE

Highlights of the Visit to the University of Kuopio, Finland

1985 – 1986

Jean Church and I arrived in Frankfurt, Germany, on August 26, 1985. Finnair took us to Helsinki, Finland, and after a two-hour wait for connections we were off to Kuopio. What a beautiful setting.

We were met at the plane and taken to a hotel for a couple of nights (Hotel Iavonia); our apartment would be available in a couple of days. It was a lovely bright apartment with two bedrooms and a cleaning lady who was a delightful young lady.

Rather than review each day, may I highlight a few?

August 30	Taken through Soko's to pick up basic groceries.
August 31	Picked up by Mr. and Mrs. Vuorikari for a garden party invited by Sirkka Sinkkonen.
September 3	Taken to bank by Sirkka Lauri and given tour of city.
September 5	Invited to music concert by Sirkka Sinkkonen and attended a beautiful program – the auditorium was so

beautiful – pale blue leather seats, light wood for seats and floor – just elegant. Outstanding music for program.

September 10   Kaisa Krause took me over to be welcomed by Rector Juhani Karja. Plans for a newspaper interview were postponed. We were served coffee and had a lovely visit in English.

Telephone hook-up was made in our apartment – everyone very happy – however, neither Jean nor I speak Finnish. My adorable and capable secretary, Pirrko Mikkanen, phonetically helped me so much. However, when I requested a taxi, I could hear the ladies at the other end snickering at my pronunciation!

September 24   Met faculty at full faculty meeting – all so very friendly and eager to help us in anything we might need.

September 27   Taught Class – Doctoral Programs in the USA, Their Similarities and Differences – to doctoral students.

October 7   Taught Class – Characteristics of Nursing Research Today – Trends and Changes – to master's students.

October 8   Addressed faculty meeting on nursing and nursing science.

October 9   8 a.m. presented my own research to Faculty and some students in coffee room.

October 11   Counseling of individual doctoral students.

October 13   At the request of the University of Kuopio, went to Helsinki.

October 14   Taught class – Developing a Research Problem – Master's Students.

	Met with Nursing Club in the evening: Maija Souveitula.
October 15	Met with Parva Huopalakt in offices of the Foundation of Nursing Education.
October 16	Returned to Kuopio.
October 18	Taught Class: University of Minnesota Doctoral Program and Nursing Resource Center – doctoral students attended discussion meeting of Reunion of Sisters with Professor Osma Hanninen, Sirkka Sirkkonan, cultural specialist, Eila Heikkila (American Embassy) and Mrs. Rose-Maria Crockett, Cutural Attaché, Embassy of the United States of America. Lunch was with Rector Jukane Kaaja.
October 20	Invited to Sirkka Sinkkonen's home for a dinner. Met her adorable daughter Sari.
November 4	Met with nursing group to start developing nursing's objectives for the elderly interdisciplinary study. Invited to lunch with Eine Laakonen.
November 5	Meeting of Elderly Interdisciplinary Research Planning Team.
November 6	Pastry brought to apartment by faculty member (8:30 a.m.); roses and other flowers brought to office as a thank you from faculty member for research counseling.
November 7	TV put in apartment.
November 8	<u>Taught Class</u> – Use of Theory in Nursing Research – Doctoral Students.
	Counseled doctoral student in her research.

	Taught Class – Application of Nursing Research to the Clinical Setting - Master's Students.
November 11	Counseling doctoral student (faculty) research.
November 12	Counseling doctoral student (faculty) research.
November 14	Meeting of Elderly Interdisciplinary Research Planning Team

Administration: Juhanne Nikkila

Dentistry: Juiga Palin – Polakae (who also looked after Jean's tooth!)

Medicine: Onni Siitonen

Nursing: Kaisa Krause, Sirkka Lauri, Pirkko Mikkanen, Sirkka Sinkkonen

Nutrition: Eine Laakkonen

Social Pharmacy: Hanne Enuld

The following discussions were in English. As before, the group continued in Finnish to further refine the project – statement of problem, the objectives, overall design and theoretical base were developed in the earlier meetings.

November 18	Counseling doctoral student (faculty) research.
November 19	Tour of hospital arranged by Sirkka Lauri.
November 20	Interview with Eila Ollikainen, journalist with *Savon Sanamat*.

November 21	Presentation of my research – Continuity of Care of Elderly at Home – at the Sosiaaligerontologian Symposium in Jyväskylä.
	There were around 2,000 present.
	After the meeting we were all invited to attend their sauna – my ears perked up! Of course, I was told, there's a sauna for women and one for men. I said – great, we're going home – and we did!
November 23	A delightful family day with Sirkka – Liisa and her family – driven around Kuopio at night to see the lights.
November 26	Meeting with Interdisciplinary Planning Team.
November 27	Research Guidance with Licentiate student (faculty).
December 2	Meeting with Interdisciplinary Planning Team.
December 3	Christmas Party at Sirkka Lauri's home.
December 6	Luncheon celebration of Independence Day with Eine Laakkonen.
December 10	Meeting with Interdisciplinary Planning Team. Our final coffee party – and Good-bye.
December 14	Leave for home.

What a joy to be working with nursing scholars who were together in growth and knowledge and in a collegial relationship. It was such a pleasure! I trust I was helpful, and I know I learned and respected very highly your commitment and hard work to improve the nursing discipline.

Each of you is making a major contribution to nursing and to each other.

Thank you for the privilege of being with you.

In reviewing your letter of March 26, 1985, I hope I have fulfilled your hopes and expectations. The teaching and research consultation I have done. The added interdisciplinary research was an opportunity for each of us. Thank you to the Science Foundation of Finland.

There is only one thing I did not include, and that was my excellent visit to the University of Tampere. The train ride was good too! Electric.

I am so thankful to each of you. And truly appreciated the coffee party and beautiful Seropkook (which many of my friends have enjoyed envisioning while listening to how wonderful you are).

Before I go on a visit to a new setting I read, think, and try to feel the setting – before I leave home. Often a poem comes forth.

May I share the poem for you – to you? (Which I did say at our Coffee Party.)

My Neighbours in Kuopio

If my neighbour needed a cup of sugar,
I would give it to her;
But what if she needed a friend?

If my neighbour needed bread,
I would bake it for her;
But what if she needed hope?

If my neighbour needed shoes,
I would provide them for her;
But what if she needed compassion?

If my neighbour needed water,
I would dig him a well;
But what if he needed a sense of worth?

Please, grant me the wisdom
To give my neighbours
What they really need, AND
Let me have the courage to give of myself.

—Floris E. King
August 1985

I know you will be anxious to learn the results of the study. A book has been written and published by the Kuopion Yliopiston Julkuisrija Publications of the University of Kuopio.

Yhteiskuntatietest (Social Sciences)
Tilastotja Belvitykser (Statistics and Review) 2/1988
Sirkka Lauri (Toim)

VANHUUDEN KOKEMINEN KUOPISSA
(TERVEYDENHUOIION HAIION IAITOS
KUOPION YIIOPISTO
KUOPIO 1988)

My copy has been signed, which I treasure.

As this was one of the first comprehensive studies of the elderly in Finland, focusing on social dimensions of aging and the meaning of the aging of population to society, a survey design was selected and each discipline developed a questionnaire related to their specialty concerns. The purpose of this research was to get an inclusive picture and opinions of the life situations, state of health and different functions of people over 70 years old living in Kuopio. (I am quoting from an extensive English report by Sirkka Lauri, who I most appreciate and respect.)

The local government of Kuopio was enlisted in drawing a sample of seniors.

Summary of a Summary Report
Prepared by Sirkka Lauri (Permission Granted)
1985 – 1986

In Kuopio, as in Finland, the population is getting older. This is especially so over 75 years old. There is a need of knowledge of their way of life and their problems in order to plan different services and understandings.

There are some weaknesses in social gerontologic basic research: examining social dimensions of aging and meaning of aging population to society.

Study
Interdisciplinary Finnish Study
On
Experiencing Old Age in Kuopio, Finland

The target population for research was all over 70 years old people in Kuopio who lived at home on the first of January, 1986. All together there were 5,660. From this population were chosen 10 individual samples that came to be 566 persons. The sample was made in the planning department of Kuopio city council in two phases. In the first phase were sampled people from 70 to 79 years and in the second phase, 80 years old people and older. The size of the sample was 339 after the dead and persons in institutions were taken away.

Men and Women Together: 566

The Questionnaires were tested by home visits, prior to them being prepared for mailing to the 566 folks.

There was an excellent return of 80% (435).

For mailed surveys, in the U.S., we consider 65 to 70% a very good reply.

The material was collected by post in two phases. Inquiry was sent to 70-79 years old in June 1986, and 80 years old or older in September 1986. The repetition inquiry was sent to both age groups in October/November 1986. There was no answering time set in the form, all forms arrived before the tenth of December 1986.

The age distribution of the old people answering the questionnaire was 44% who were under 75 years old and 23% 80 years old and older.

Much detail was collected and documented in the report and the analysis.

Old people's health can be observed from two points of view - point of disease, and in regard to functional model health – a state of well being. Probably old people look on their health mostly through their functionality. Many of us as we get older look toward functionality – much more optimistic than the medical model.

Consequently the analysis of the data was done as follows:

Need of Services and Receiving Help

- Background Variables and Social Network
- Physical Functionality
- Experiencing Life
- Situation
- Social Functionality
- Experiencing Health
- Health Behavior and Experiencing
- Influencing Possibilities

Using this format the data were organized and analyzed by the following scholars (<u>Students in the different disciplines also participated</u>):

- 2 students from Nutrition and Eating received their degrees as reported by Eini Laakkonen, which is a wonderful way for students to learn.
- I understand there were others too, but presently I don't know of them. Sorry about that – think this learning is just so great.
- Pirkko Mikkanen wrote up the details of the research methods and materials; Pirkko (my dear secretary while I was there) also wrote up the State of Health, Functionality and Receiving Help Experienced by Old People.
- Tuija Palen-Palokas wrote about Old People's Health of Mouth and Need of Health Services for Mouth.
- Eini Laakonen and student Anja Karinpaa presented Old People's Nutrition and Eating (Good for you, Anja Karinpaa).
- Hannes Enlund reported on Old People's Use of Medicine
- Sirkka Sinkkonen and Juhani Nikkila wrote about Old People's Attitudes and Influencing Efforts to Social and Health Politics on Municipal Level (Good for you, Juhani Nikkila).
- Kaisa Krause wrote on Old People's Satisfaction with their Life Direction.
- Sirkka Lauri, along with everything else, wrote the Summary and Discussion.

You are all so very Special -
Thank you for a Research Study Well Done.

THIRTEEN

Return to the University of Minnesota School of Nursing

1986 - 1991

*R*eturned to my home – most appreciative to have my condo. Then I learned Mother was dying of esophageal cancer, and had six months to live. I requested a six month leave of absence without pay from Dean Fahy.

I was refused as I was told no one else could teach the Doctoral Research – and these students needed it <u>right then</u>. With the students I arranged every third weekend to be a long weekend to be with Mother. Physically, mentally, and emotionally I was devastated. But for Mother I did my best. I arranged home care, as that's what she wanted. Every third Friday afternoon, I flew to Regina to be met by a friend. After an hour on the highway I would arrive home. Mother was in bed but I lay beside her so she knew I was there. Soon I went to bed. I was with her until Monday afternoon and returned to Minneapolis. It was so hard to leave her. The last two weeks she was in hospital. I had special nurses with her – but I should have been there.

I wanted so badly to retire early. I did.

With the trunk of my car filled up, I returned on a Sunday, picked up my door name plate and quietly drove around Lake of the Isles and Lake Harriet three times and peacefully went home. I had done all I could.

After Mother's death, I invited three Finnish students, arranged by the University of Minnesota International Students Organization, to Christmas dinner each year for six years. What wonderful people. I love them. As soon as they arrived, I had them phone their home. When I learned their names, I would write them to alert their family at home so the family would be awaiting their call.

—Kiitos
(Thank you)

FOURTEEN

A Few Concluding Moments of Thought and Thank You

Throughout my journey, I have met so many wonderful and kind people. In this story I have thanked many. So many more need thanks as well – all of whom I could not possibly mention. I am most appreciative of you all. Thank you.

A few I would like to give special recognition to: (I know you would like to know them too.)

- Judge John (Jack) Guy and Gail, my cousins in Winnipeg, who gave me a beautiful silver-covered book with blank pages plus a silver photograph album with blank photographic page holders. I asked them what this was for –"to write the story of your life." So with a few gentle but firm pushes, here I am! Thank you Jack and Gail – you are special.
- My dear friend Heather Mitchell, who immediately wanted to work with me on my "Story" with her excellent computer skills and special knowledge of what the computer could do, which were all pluses. But most of all was her love and commitment to work with me. You are special in so many ways, my dear one. Being in Etobicoke, Canada, Heather worked it all out. Thank you so much Heather, dear one.

- Ruth Weise is a special friend – not only with a loving spirit but a friend through and through. The University at Rochester perhaps understands the overall love the students have for Ruth who committed a scholarly effort for teaching and learning in Rochester for two full quarters a year for ten years on the Theories of Nursing, the Discipline of Nursing, etc. I joined her on her trips for only two years during the winter quarter. She picked me up at my home and brought me back at her insistence – and it was COLD. Some weeks the roads were mighty ICY, but Ruth kept going, slow and steady. I am not sure if anyone thanked her for her encouragement to have a graduate program in Rochester – but I do. Her encouragement was mostly from the students – her true love.
- Dee and Beth (Dianna I.M. Summich and Ethel E. Reaburn) provided loving care for Mother and her suite, which was well cared for. In all weather, I was met at the Regina airport and driven back and forth. Two genuine, darling friends of the family. And now, with Mother's passing, they continue to extend their love to me – birthdays, long telephone calls, keeping me up to date of happenings in Town and Country – which means so much to me. They are great cat lovers, and I have pictures of their cats when they were alive. Now they have a cat given to them by the veterinarian who received it after it was hit on the road as a kitten. He just knew Beth and Dee would look after it. Indeed, they have. The cat now "permits" Beth and Dee to live with her! With the cat's head damage, she requires special care and much patience – and based on the loving pictures I receive, she is getting it!
- There are so many more, please forgive me for not including you. But there is one dear soul who hunted for me for years, and finally through the Internet, her husband found me. I received a telephone call from Toronto. It was Dorothy Eagan, who is now the wife of Pastor Kenneth Moon and calls herself Dotti. She said

she just had to see me. On their way home from Florida, they could change their flight so there would be a four-hour stopover in Minneapolis, if it was alright with me! Obviously the hours went quickly by. What a joyous reunion which continues to grow on and on. She is a darling and so is Ken. When she phones, she asks, "How is my music teacher?" Being neighbors in Toronto, the Eagans would hear me practicing and had insisted I take Dorothy as a student! I learned that she kept all the books I wrote in with the "stars," and her three daughters (one a musician) learned how to play "as her teacher taught her." Oh my, what a thrill to be rejoined with Dotti, who calls frequently now. It's like old times when we get together. She prepared a scrapbook for me to show her playing for choirs, concerts, etc. – a complete joy. Thank you Dotti and Pastor Ken.

Thank You To All

Thank you God, for bringing me this far
This far in faith
This far in love
This far in courage.

I could not have made this journey
Without your strength
Without your guidance
Without your love.

But I want to go further, God,
To be more loving
To be more courageous
To be – more…

—Floris E. King
2008

Very Best Wishes to
Dean Connie Delaney
Happy Centennial
School of Nursing, University of Minnesota

Article #1

King, Floris E. First National Conference of Research in Nursing Practice
Ottawa, 1971
Department of National Health and Welfare
Grant Number 610-22-1XX

SCHOLARLY PURSUIT OF EXCELLENCE:
DOCTORAL EDUCATION IN NURSING

Floris E. King
Professor, School of Nursing
University of Minnesota

Doctoral education is the scholarly pursuit of excellence in a defined discipline. Doctorial education in nursing provides an opportunity for nurses to study, test and evolve theories, to conduct research, and then to translate theoretical concepts and research findings into care of clients and patients.

To discuss this scholarly pursuit of excellence, the following areas will be reviewed: the growth of doctoral programs in nursing, development of nursing science, and finally, the continued growth of scholarly excellence in nursing.

Growth of Doctoral Education Programs in Nursing

Doctoral education in nursing has evolved with the development of the discipline. Nursing began as a practice-oriented discipline consisting of technically trained apprentices. It slowly eased into academia and professional education by incorporating relevant knowledge from the arts and sciences, by conducting research on practice, and by developing theory which could be translated into practice. Such progress was not without resistance:

> *The education of nurses in an academic setting, however, was not encouraged due to the fear by some health-related groups that nurses would become too knowledgeable and hospital might suffer an economic loss in its dependable source of workers needed to staff the agency.*[1]

As early as 1923, the Goldmark Report advocated moving the control of nursing education from hospitals to institutions of higher learning.[2] That report and many others that followed had little impact. It was not until the end of World War II when large numbers of nurses eligible for G.I. benefits enrolled in colleges and universities, that the growth of school of nursing and institutions of higher education began to move forward. Consequently, this expansion of university-based undergraduate programs for nurses stimulated a greater need for graduate level studies designed to prepare nurses for teaching or administrative roles. As a result, master's level programs in nursing were established or expanded in every region of the United States and Canada during the decade of the 1950s.[3]

During this period, nurses began to enroll in a wide variety of doctoral programs – in education, natural and social sciences. The Nurse Scientist Training Act supported doctoral programs offering the doctorate of philosophy in the health, the natural and the behavioral sciences related to nursing. Matarazzo and Abdellah stated this development very succinctly:

First generation nurse scientists sought their doctoral training predominately in education and the behavioral and social sciences. A few pursued the biological sciences. More recently, doctoral training in the clinical

---

[1] Guinee, Kathleen K. *The Professional Nurse: Orientation, Roles and Responsibilities.* London, Ontario: MacMillan Company, 1970.

[2] Goldsmith, Josephine. *Nursing and Nursing Education in the U.S.A.* New York: MacMillan Company, 1923.

[3] Dr. Floris King organized the first National Conference on Research in Nursing Practice held in Ottawa in February, 1971. She was at the time on faculty at the University of British Columbia.

specialties has produced clinical nurse specialists. These kinds and combinations of training have produced hybrid teachers (second generations). Such individuals are nurses, but they are also scientists and clinical specialists. From these programs will come the third generation, teachers of Ph.D. in nursing.[4]

Cleland also noted the importance of these initial academic steps:

Women are considerably more welcome in academia today... In fact, with the current uneasiness about too many people with doctorates, the qualified nurse applicant is especially attractive, because job placement in nursing is not a problem. In addition, nurses have proven themselves as able student who also possess east access to the health care system for research purposes.[5]

Readiness for doctoral educational growth is reflected in many ways. Job requirements are demanding that nurses doctoral preparation in the roles of educator, administrator, research or clinician.[6] Nurse scholars, in whatever role, seek to study behavioral and physiological phenomena that would add or validate previous knowledge about human phenomena, and thereby contribute to theory development relevant to nursing practice.

Conferences and seminars have been conducted to further support doctoral education growth in Canada and the United States. For example, Canada's first National Conference on Research in Nursing Practice was held in Ottawa, February 16-18, 1971 with over 300 present. This unique conference focused on research in nursing practice, essential to doctoral education.[7] The Kellogg National Seminar on Doctoral Preparation for Canadian

---

4   Matarazzo, Joseph d. and Abdellah, Fay. "Doctoral Education for nurses in the United State," Nursing Research.20:5: 404-414, September-October, 1971.
5   Cleland, Virginia. "Developing a Doctoral Program," *Nursing Outlook*. 24:10:631-635, October 1976.
6   National League for Nursing. *Doctoral Programs in Nursing, 1979-1980*. NLN Publication No. 15-1448, New York: NLN, 1979
7   King, Floris E. *First National Conference on Research in Nursing Practice*. Ottawa, 1971. Report: Department of National Health and Welfare, Grant number 610-22-1.

Nurses, held in 1978, also provided much impetus for the consideration of developing doctoral education in Canada for nurses.[8]

The type of doctoral preparation that is considered, is significant in directing the evolution of scientific systems. Nursing science needs persons with doctoral education in nursing; there is also a need for doctorally-prepared persons in all nursing-related disciplines. However, the critical need at the doctoral level is not the area of preparation but the commitment to develop science in nursing.

Development of Nursing Science

The ultimate goal of nursing's scholarly pursuit of excellence is the development of nursing science. There are several stages to this scientific development.

Science is an attempt to organize experience. Frank states:

> *"Science advances through the formulation of a body of postulates and assumptions, a conceptual framework… (which) provides a coherent, internally unified way of thinking about the event and processes in each discipline for which it is relevant. This approach fosters the conception of science as a systematic and never ending endeavour…"*[9]

Frank's conceptualization suggests that science is a product that advances, as well as the process by which it evolves.

Kuhn, in *The Structure of Scientific Revolutions*[10] states that the early stage of scientific development is the pre-paradigm stage. This is characterized by divergent schools of thought which, although addressing the range of phenomena, usually describe and interpret these phenomena in different ways.

---

8   Stinson, Shirley. *Kellogg National Seminar on Doctoral Preparation for Canadian Nurses*. Ottawa: Canadian Nurses Association, 1979.
9   Frank, L.K. "Science as Communication Process," *Main Currents of Modern Thought.."* 25:2 November-December, 1968.
10 Kuhn, T. *The Structure of Scientific Revolution*. 2nd ed. Chicago: University of Chicago Press, 1970.

Through accumulation of knowledge, testing and retesting, a metaparadigm evolves. This is considered the broadest consensus within the discipline. In general, the metaparadigm or prevailing paradigm: 1) is accepted by most members of the discipline, 2) serves as a way of organizing perceptions, 3) defines what entities are of interest, 4) tells the scientists where to find these entities, 5) tells them what to expect, 6) tells them how to study them.

Although the period of theory development in a discipline is characterized by ambiguity and uncertainty, nurse scientists can help built the knowledge base that will help formulation an acceptable paradigm. They can do this by being well informed in a substantive area and participating actively in both theory construction and research.[11]

To select only one paradigm for the discipline of nursing is questionable. This may be restrictive. The body of knowledge of nursing science must ultimately withstand the repeated investigation of theoretically-based problems. In this way knowledge is redefined as research results accumulate. Several paradigms will evolve.

Theoretical formulations are already evolving within the discipline. A sample of related discipline theories used in nursing research today include: the disengagement theory, cognitive dissonance theory, theory of status consistency theory, systems theory, communication theory, self-actualization theory, and grief and loss theory. Some select nursing theories include the following:

- Roy (1976): Man, as a holistic being in constant interaction with the environment, adapts through mechanisms that manifest themselves through adaptive modes: physiological, self-concept, role function, and interdependence.
- Orem (1978, 1980): Individuals have self-care that facilitates self-care health practices. If this agency is insufficient to meet self-care demands, then self-care limitations occur that legitimate a relationship with a nurse.

---

11 Hardy, Margaret E. "Perspectives on Nursing Theory," *Advances in Nursing Science.* 1:1:37048, October, 1978.

- King (1971, 1978): Man operates in social systems through communication in terms of perception that affect his health.
- Paterson and Zderad (1976): Nursing is an intersubjective transaction that occurs in "the between" of the nurse-nursed and through which nurturance occurs.
- Johnson (1974): Man is a behavioral system composed of seven subsystems. If the behavioral system is functioning effectively (ineffectively) in meeting subsystem goals, then the system is in balance (imbalance).
- Rogers (1970, 1978): The life processes are unidirectional along the space-time continuum where continuous interactions between man and environment are characterized by wave patterns.

There is an interrelatedness of theory and experience. The discipline includes nurses who are clearly "doers" or practitioners. The discipline must also include scientists dedicated to generating knowledge. Nursing practice and nursing science are not antithetical – each depends on the other. Doctoral education provides the bridge.

The Continued Growth of Excellence in Nursing

The continued growth of excellence evolves from the practice of nursing, the research which is conducted on nursing phenomena and their interrelationships, and the rigorous testing for developing theories in nursing. The fruits of the refinement of nursing science is not only reflected in – but actually enjoyed and further tested in nursing practice. This organization of postulates and assumptions in a systematic structure is continuously tested as it relates to the real world of practice. Doctoral education provides the level of scholarly endeavor toward this pursuit of excellence. As Ralph Waldo Emerson stated: "The office of the scholar is to cheer, and guide men by showing them the facts amidst appearance."[12]

---

12 Emerson, Ralph Waldo. *The complete Essays and Other Writings of Ralph Waldo Emerson*. New York: The Modern Library, 1950. p 55.

Article #2

The Formative Years of the Author, 1927-1948

I was born June 27, 1927, in my grandparents' home (Jack and Evelyn Guy) in Caron, Saskatchewan – 21 miles west of Moose Jaw. Nurse Moody, a nurse-midwife from England who had been with Mother from her sixth month of pregnancy, delivered me. The doctor was in the country delivering another baby and was not available.

I was told many times by Mother that, when Nurse Moody put me to her breast, I seized it, and like a vice, I refused to let go. With Mother screaming, Nurse Moody had to hold my little nose until I let go. As for taking a bottle, I gulped that down every time. I stayed a while with my grandparents.

My mother and father were both in the church choir. As Mother didn't "show" until late in the sixth month, the choir called me the "Surprise Baby." During church services, as an infant, I remained in my carriage at the back of the church. Mother said there was always someone at the back who would attend to me, but I seldom cried. When I was old enough to sit up, my father had me beside him in the choir. He said I had a good tenor voice!

As I was at Nanna and Papa's home frequently, Nanna kept telling Mother I didn't go to sleep when she rocked me. This Nanna could not understand. Mother told her that she never rocked me – she would just put me down, and I would go to sleep!

There are a few happenings Mother told me about, but many of my remembrances were quite happy.

My father and I went on many walks together. When I could sit up, he pulled me in the wooden wagon with a big pillow. So if I got tired, I would just lie down and sleep.

Later, our walks were full of topics. We would look and listen to the birds, the chirping of the crickets, and the clop of horses going by. Later, we would pretend we were something, such as a robin, and try to follow the life of a robin, what it did. Another pretending included being a window pane and observing all the windows on our walk – small, large, broken, clean, dirty. We'd guess if there were more dirty or clean and theorize how did a window get cleaned away up high. We would go to the church and discuss why it had such beautiful windows. Sometimes we were a pair of shoes and would discuss the differences on all the shoes people wore. This was always great fun. Soon, I was asked who we would be on our journey today!

Dad had a beautiful way with children. He loved all the children in the neighborhood. He even went out and played ball with them.

Mother, Dad and I had lovely get-togethers before bedtime. Mother would play songs and hymns on the piano, and we would all sing. The cat would disappear (tenor really upset him) – he was not musically inclined! It surprised both Mom and Dad when I would start singing the right song after just a couple of notes on the piano were played. I just knew what was coming!

By age three, I was starting to "play at" the piano; I just loved picking out the different beautiful melodies. The bass could be arranged so the melody was either happy or sad. A remarkable find! At three, I made my first stage appearance – standing on a chair on the stage of a large hall at a Mother's Day Concert, with Mother at the piano! Mother said that, even at the very back of the hall, not only could everyone see me; they also heard every word and every note! I liked it too!

I won several Music Festival Honors. Mrs. Carter, who was so funny with children, taught me my first lessons. She told Mother and Dad that I needed a professional musician, that she could no longer keep up to me.

My father, Mother, and I visited the Anglican Boarding School in Regina, Saskatchewan, called Qu'Appelle Diocesan Girls School. They wore uniforms and had a music teacher, Sister Cecelia, who smiled and took my hand. Sister had been with Mona Bates, Canada's top pianist. Well, I was ready!

Doris Connick was my roommate all the way through to grade twelve. A better person you could never meet. We were as one. Doris became a nurse anesthesiologist and did her practice in rural areas in Saskatchewan and North Dakota. She was a most committed human being. Sadly, she did not live long; she died of cancer. I feel part of me is carrying on for her.

I worked hard at school and music and loved every minute. Sister Cecelia's studio was just down the hall from the room I shared with Doris. It seemed right that we were so close. Sister was wonderful. She knew so much and had fun with me trying out different things. Also at times, she insisted I go for a walk with her around a near lake; she wanted me to get fresh air and exercise. I introduced her to some of Dad's games when we were walking! She came up with some great topics to consider.

I gave recitals in the Darke Hall auditorium and was even invited to play on the radio. Now, that was an event. Even Mother, Dad, and Sister Cecelia were invited to that.

After church at the cathedral in downtown Regina, on Sunday, Sister Cecelia and I had our dinner privately together in the Sisters' Lounge so we could listen to the live New York Symphony Program on the radio. I thought heaven must be like that!

I worked very hard, and arrangements were made with the University of Toronto for me to get the four-year courses under the supervision of Sister Cecelia. A professor from the University would come out from Toronto to evaluate my performance on the piano.

My studies went very well; my schedule was well planned.

Every summer I went to Nanna and Papa's home – what a beautiful relaxing time. Some summers Patsy Keeler (my chum since we were three years of age) was invited to join us. Patsy and I explored all the bush lands and countryside we could get to! There was only one rule in the household:

- If we wanted to stay up to 10 p.m. (Nanna and Papa had many wonderful visitors who told great tales together – and we didn't want to miss them!) we had to take an afternoon nap from 2 to 4.
- Otherwise we went to bed at 8:00 p.m.

Some choice! We selected the former!

Once, Nanna broke the rule. Our house was next door to the church, and one afternoon there was a wedding. Up came Nanna to wake us and help us dress, and then she took us to the back of the church to watch the wedding. We thought that was great!

Mother and Dad went to Vancouver every summer. I always declined to join them. I had gone a couple of times – and it was lovely seeing some of the things – but I always had to be dressed up. It was better at Nanna's!

So after the final four years (two of which I was named a prefect of the school with certain responsibilities; but these were very, very limited, as I had a full load), I graduated with honours for Solo Performers in Music from the University of Toronto, and First Class Honours in eight high school courses – what was going to be next? I was sad leaving the school and all the wonderful sisters. It was home.

With Sister Cecelia's guidance and assistance, Sister Cecelia, Mother and I took off to Toronto to meet with Mona Bates. I didn't realize going in, but this was a test to see if Mona Bates would take me. She was only taking four to six students at the time. I played a couple of selections she asked for; we did some harmony and ear exercises together; and we talked some.

The sum of it all was – she was delighted to take me.

Then what?

Arrangements were made for me to live in a Ladies Professorial Hall – quite an elegant spot. It was just one and a half blocks from Mona Bates, and half a block from a music hall where Dad rented a room for me to practice. This I did daily from 9-12 and 1-4, except for Sunday. Mona Bates required this commitment, as every two weeks I had to learn a new selection in order to get my repertoire up. Also, I played in her private recital in her studio with others. Her studio was magnificent – her home being a large, elegant stone house. One end of the studio had two large Steinway pianos next to each other – one for her, and the other for a student. The other end of the studio had a large fireplace and several large, comfortable chairs. It was most impressive. I wished we had talked more. But a lesson consisted of me playing what I had learned that week with her stopping me at times to play a section as she wanted it to be played. She was so brilliant, sitting there wearing her long velvet gowns. The dark green one I particularly liked, but I didn't have much time to really look at it. It was all business. No talking.

It was an excellent learning experience, BUT – I was all alone. The other ladies in the residence were older and socialized mostly with others in their own professions. I wasn't even sure who to eat with.

I gave a Sunday concert there that was well attended and appreciated. I was still the kid on the block. I tried walking outside in the beautiful grounds which also had a tennis court, but I couldn't see the sky – how I missed seeing the prairie horizon and sunsets. I felt literally scared and wondered how long I could hang on.

Life in the City

Herein the city,
Many people milling 'round
They come and go –
The other not known –
Unfound.

A friend may come along the way
With inner beauty glow
A mind, a sense,
A feel – intense
Not so.

To live this life one must have

An inner life alone,
To think, to feel
To pray, reveal –
A "home."

This "home" must be on solid ground,
Within one's own abode,
My thoughts and songs –
Where one belongs –
Now.

Not in the life of the city,
For here is too much strife,
The outside is cold –
No more to hold –
The pulse of life.

—Floris E. King

Soon professional piano concert tours were to come. I began to wonder how long I was going to be able to hold on. I was not a good traveler, and the schedule was rigorous – no rest days.

Then came Father to see how I was doing. He took one look at me and said, "You are too alone here. It is time we had a home here." He bought a house in Toronto, one with two fireplaces! I loved them. I began to breathe again – oh, neighbors. They heard me practicing, of course, and along came neighbors' children who wanted me to teach them to play the piano. Three stood out – Dorothy, Larry, and Marguerite. (I mention the story of Dorothy [Dotti] in the last chapter of the book.) I loved them all.

So with three tours with concerts to keep up, I was very busy again.

Finally, just before the fourth tour, I told Mona Bates, I was unable to take the tour and needed to think about continuing with music. Well! My parents were notified. This indeed was a tragedy for Mother, who enjoyed the tours, traveling, social gatherings. I felt so badly for everyone, but as much as I loved the performances themselves, I knew I just could not do any more.

I called my father, and he came. I explained the whole situation. He said he understood and said I must do what I wanted to do. He asked if I'd had time to think through what was really right for me. I said I had – I wanted to take the beautiful essence of the discipline of music and re-invent it, to develop this into caring for people – medicine or nursing. I wanted to observe and visit with doctors and nurses in hospitals, public health care, the Victorian Order of Nurses and clinics, and then I would decide.

Dad said, "Do it. Let me know how I can help."

Appendix A

Nursing Model of Research

- Continuity of Care of — — — — — — — —
- Interdisciplinary of Care of — — — — — — —
- Humaness of Care of — — — — — — — —

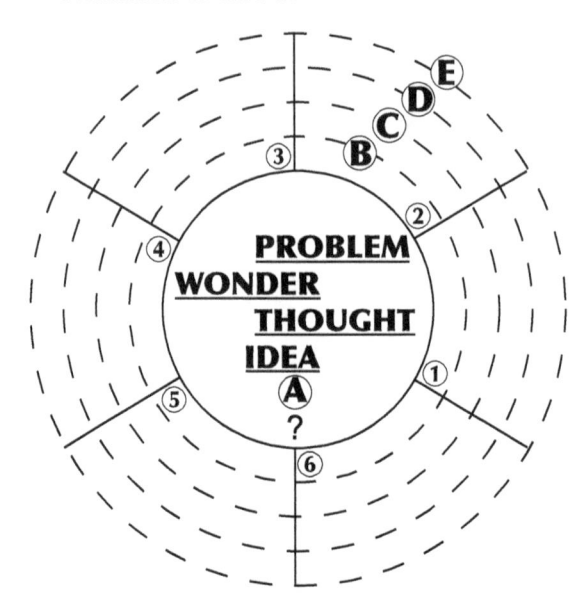

Ⓐ Special Preparation for Study – Research

Ph. D. Preparation
M.D. Preparation
P.T. Preparation
B. S. C. N. Preparation
D. N. S. Preparation
Psychologist Preparation
Psychiatrist Preparation
Spiritualist (Pastor) Preparation
Administration Preparation
Dentistry Preparation
Statistician Preparation
Computer Science Preparation

Select appropriate team members re: Problem, Needs, Thought, Idea,?

Ⓑ Pt./Family/Friends/Community Care
Ⓒ Pt./Basic Care – ex. yearly physical
Ⓓ Pt./Episodic Illness
Ⓔ Pt./Long-Term Care

} All age groups

Examples

1. More understanding of a problem structure.
2. How is a specific treatment more problematic/helpful.
3. Specific outcomes as seen by the patient; patients perceptions as compared with _____.
4. Want to know more about _____.
5. As a group want to understand more about _____.
6. Elderly/other age group coping/not coping with _____.

Floris E. King Ph. D.
1972 ©

Appendix B

ARTICLE

Floris E. King Ph.D., RN Professor and Research Officer, School of Nursing, University of Minnesota,

Judy Figge RN Director and Chief Executive Officer, Austin Management Corporation and

Patricia Harman RN MS Research Assistant, Graduate Program in Nursing, University of Minnesota

The elderly coping at home:
a study of continuity of nursing care

Accepted for publication 1 May 1985

The Challenge of Nursing

The challenge of nursing today is to meet the growing complexity of the care needs of the ageing. Each of us grows older every day. According to Cowgill (1967) there is no universally accepted criterion as to when old age begins. Its definition tends to vary geographically, temporarily, and from one person to another. In the United States the arbitrary age is 65, which is the accepted age for eligibility for Social Security benefits, as well as private retirement and annuity programs (Aiken 1978, Shanas and Maddox 1976). Many elderly people attempt to slow down or camouflage the effects of ageing, while others attempt to conceal their age not only from others but even from themselves.

By the end of 1980 there were more than 26 million people over the age of 65 in the United States, which accounted for 11% of the total population. By 1990, it is projected that 12%, and by 2000, 13% of the population will be over 65 years of age. By 2030, one out of every four will be 60 or older (Pegels, 1981). The elderly are living longer, and the very old elderly (75 years and above) are the most rapidly growing part of the population. Consequently, there are more dependent elderly to care for than ever before. Besides, families are smaller in size, often living geographically apart from the elderly, in smaller homes and apartments, and are more likely to be employed than at home. Consequently, there is decreased family care for the elderly.

Most of the health problems in older age-groups come from chronic rather than acute conditions, with heart disease, arthritis and chronic rheumatism being the most frequent chronic conditions (Health Care Financing Administration 1981). Although most people aged 65 and older have chronic conditions but are not functionally impaired, the probability of suffering from an accumulation of chronic conditions rises precipitously with age. More than half of the population aged 85 experience major limitations in their activities of daily living (Shanas & Maddox 1976). Public health (home health) nurses have traditionally functioned relatively independently with physician collaboration in patients' homes:

...where they have assessed problems of individuals and families treated minor illnesses, referred patients to social service agencies and organizations, given advice and counsel to promote health and prevent illness, supervised pregnant women and worked with community action programs.

Nursing Outlook 1972

Areas of functioning of the elderly Figure 1

	Biological	Ageing Process	Biological	
	Individual	Increase in Numbers; Developmental level	Individual	
Familial	• Lives with family • Intergenerational • Larger Homes		• Family not near • Lives alone- • Apartments • Small homes	Familial
Sociocultural	• Community activities centered around family		• Lack of social contacts • Transportation problems • Social groups attempts to meet social needs	Sociocultural
Health/illness Care	• Personal Family care • General care • Care given by family		• Group, social care • High cost • Negative Attitudes to elderly • Specialized care • Nursing homes	Health/illness Care
	Before 1960		After 1960	

Mundinger (1983) identified two distinct elderly populations who can benefit from home care: (a) those who have been hospitalized with an acute episode of illness or disability and subsequently require convalescent health care outside the institution; and (b) those who have not been institutionalized but are at risk for such placement because of their deteriorating health or waning self-care abilities.

This study addresses the first population group for the purposes of adding to the knowledge base of nursing care of the elderly who have been discharged from hospital to home. What is the relationship between coping levels of the elderly at home with certainty/uncertainty scores, perceived levels of health, and perceived satisfaction with the nursing care services?

In summary. Figure 1 presents the change in biological, individual, familial, sociocultural, and health/illness care areas which affect the functioning of the elderly. An approximate date of 1960 is selected to show the before and after relationships.

Theoretical Framework

This study is based on three postulates.

Ageing is a developmental not a decremental experience

Ageing has for too long been associated with decline rather than with development, which is regarded as positive and functional for a living system (Reed 1983). Development involves a progression from generalized to the more specialized with greater levels of integration. In the early years of one's life there is both growth and development, whereas in the later years, development continues but growth slows and appears to stop (Reed 1983). Human health and functioning are integrally related to developmental phenomena.

Human development is:

1. a life-long process which continues through-out the ageing years;
2. described by multiple determinants in which the individual and context are in continual reaction;
3. influenced by the historical time in which the individual and his cohorts are living: and
4. Multi-determined and complex for any behavioral area, and is not primarily determined by age.

As people age, meaningful interactions with their environment become increasingly important for the realization of human potential

The interactions between self and the environment give meaning to the inner and physical self. Erikson's theory (1963) is significant because it explains the individual's development on the basis of encounters with the social environment throughout an eight-stage model of social growth and development. Development proceeds in a series of critical periods and a person's degree of success in passing through one stage will influence one's ability to move to the next.

If development is to progress, environmental interactions are critical. Rather than institutionalizing and isolating the elderly, meaningful environmental interactions must be enriched to enhance levels of coping with resultant feelings of well-being.

Newman's conceptual framework describes the relationship of an individual to his or her environment.

> *The individual and the environment are conceived as two open systems that are energy fields without boundaries and constantly interacting with each other. The continuous interaction between the individual and environmental energy fields is characterized by change that is both rhythmic and patterned. As these energy fields inexorably change, the individual and the environment become more complex and decrease in their*

rhythmic patterns. Consequently, a person becomes more complex with age, and ageing is viewed as a positive phenomenon of continued growth and development.

Adults are increasingly capable of transforming contradictory or conflict situations into meaningful experience

The individual continually strives toward greater order, complexity, and self-differentiation. This striving is to find and fulfill meaning with what one is coping with in regard to life events (Frankl 1969). These life events for the elderly often contain a multiplicity of pathology that have major repercussions in the psychological well-being and social interaction of the individual, and these conditions are on a continuing basis and reflect how the individual perceives his own health.

Utilizing these three postulates as the theoretical base, the relationship between levels of coping of the elderly at home was tested with the independent variables of certainty/uncertainty, perceived levels of health, and perceived support care services.

Hypotheses

Six hypotheses were formulated: (a) there is no significant relationship between levels of coping and certainty/uncertainty scores; (b) there is no significant relationship between levels of coping and perceived level of health; (c) there is no significant relationship between levels of coping and perceived support care services; (d) there is no significant relationship between levels of coping and certainty/uncertainty scores between the first and second visits; (e) there is no significant relationship between levels of coping and perceived level of health between the first and second visits; and (f) there is no significant relationship between levels of coping and perceived support care services between the first and second visits.

Definition of terms

Definitions used in this study were:

Coping

The ability to purposefully transform the present context with all its problems and contradictions into energy for development (Riegel 1975). This includes that one (a) takes pleasure from the round of activities that constitutes everyday life; (b) regards life as meaningful and accepts resolutely that which life has been; (c) feels one has succeeded in achieving one's major goals; (d) holds a positive image of one's self; and (e) maintains happy and optimistic attitudes and mood (Neugarten el al. 1961).

Certainty/uncertainty

An event is judged uncertain when it contains one or more of the following eight dimensions: (a) vagueness; (b) lack of clarity; (c) ambiguity; (d) unpredictability; (e) inconsistency; (f) probability; (g) multiple meanings; and (h) lack of information (Mishel 1982, Norton 1975). Certainty is the antithesis of uncertainty.

Self-perception (of health and of satisfaction with care)

The dynamic, conscious, continuous and active gaining of knowledge about the psychological, physical, environmental, and philosophical components of the inner self (Cambell 1980). Awareness is also used in the literature when addressing self-perception.

Continuity of home care nursing

Services furnished to an individual under the care of a physician, by staff members of a home-health care entity (home health agency, hospital or long-term care facility certified to provide home care) and managed by nurses.

Method

The study was conducted in a metropolitan area in the Midwest utilizing In Home Health Care, Inc. and its branch, In Home Services Inc. (HHC/IHC) which have been incorporated in the State of Minnesota in 1977 and 1981 respectively. The objectives of the services are to provide comprehensive, coordinated home-health nursing care 4-24 hours per day, 7 days per week to individuals and family members in their homes. Both incorporations are owned and managed by nurses. They deliver service to the seven-county metropolitan area for Medicare/Medicaid home-health nursing care visits.

The sampling procedure used in this study was purposive in nature. The subjects were 38 elderly patients (65 years of age or over) who were discharged from hospital by the physician to the care of HHC/IHS. The admission nurse of HHC/IHS notified the research office of the admission of a client to their service. A letter was sent by the HHC/IHS inviting the client to participate in the study, explaining the purpose of the study, and assuring that participation was voluntary. The investigator then telephoned the client 3-4 days following the mailing of the letter to invite the client to participate, answer questions, and to make an appointment for a home visit with the client. At the first visit, the purpose of the study was again explained and also what was expected of the participant in the study. If the client decided to participate a consent form was signed. Then the four instruments were administered, taking approximately 30 minutes. In 2-3 months the subjects were visited a second time and the instruments re-administered.

Instruments

Life Satisfaction Index A

The scale reflects the level of coping as expressed by the individual in relation to (a) takes pleasure from the round of activities that constitutes everyday life; (b) regards life as meaningful and accepts resolutely that which life has been; (c) feels has succeeded in achieving major goals; (d) holds a positive image of self; (e) maintains happy and optimistic attitudes and moods (Neugarten et al. 1961). The reliability of the scale is 0-87.

Mishel Uncertainty in Illness Scale (MUIS)

The instrument (Mishel 1982) was developed to investigate the role of uncertainty in illness and recovery. MUIS is a particularly valuable instrument in studying coping with chronic conditions. An event is judged uncertain when it contains one or more of the following eight dimension: (a) vagueness; (b) lack of clarity; (c) ambiguity; (d) unpredictability; (e) inconsistency; (f) probability; (g) multiple meanings; and (h) lack of information (Norton 1975). Certainty is the antithesis of uncertainty. The instrument possesses high reliability (0-88) and has construct and convergent validity.

Health Rating Scale and the Satisfaction with Services Scale

Both of these were self-perceived scales of 0-10 with 10 being excellent and 0 being poor.

A pilot study was conducted utilizing these instruments a year previous to this study. As a result of the pilot, the instruments were found to be reliable, valid, and practical in studying the research problem.

Results

Of the sample of 38, 3 died and 2 went to a nursing home after the first visit. The remaining 33 presented the following profile: 69.7% of the sample were women; 33.3% of the total were between the ages of 65-71 and 30.3% between 80-84, with 15.2% in the 85-89 age group; 33.3% were either married or widowed; 57.6% had an elementary school education; 60.6% lived in a house; 42.4% of the sample lived alone and 45.5% lived with 1 or 2 others; of those living with 1 or 2 others, 66.7% of these were not with the spouse; and Medicare (93.9%) was the major means of financial support.

Although this study focused on coping and not disease entities, a sample of the conditions included: COPD and esophageal stricture with Oxygen daily; radical mastectomy; pacemaker implant; diabetes; hypertension and residual right side weakness from CVA; intestinal obstruction; Shy Dragger Syndrome; triple by-pass coronary surgery; and lumbar fusion.

Table 1 presents the summary if the Pearson correlation coefficients of the independent variables and levels of coping.

For hypothesis 1, the relationship between levels of coping and certainty/uncertainty scores is significant at the P<0.001 level in the first visit, and the second visit is significant at the P<0.005 level. The null hypothesis can be rejected with confidence.

Table 1 Summary of Pearson correlation coefficients of independent variables and level of coping

Categories/indices	Level of coping
First visit	
Certainty/uncertainty	0.6129*
Perceived health	0.6548*
Perceived care	0.2583
Second visit	
Certainty/uncertainty	0.7432**
Perceived health	0.3884***
Perceived care	0.3029
Change (second visit-first visit)	
Certainty/uncertainty	0.3299
Perceived health	0.4489****
Perceived care	0.1079

*P <0.001   **P <0.005   ***P <0.05   ****P <0.01

For hypothesis 2, the relationship between the levels of coping and perceived health is significant at the $P<0.001$ level in the first visit and in the second visit is significant at the $P<0.05$ level. The null hypothesis can be rejected with confidence.

For hypothesis 3, the relationship between levels of coping and perception of care is not significant at the 0.05 level, and the nil hypothesis is accepted.

For hypothesis 4, the relationship of change between first and second visit of certainty/uncertainty (r-0.3299, $P<0.06$) to coping levels does not meet the 0.05 level of significance and the null hypothesis is accepted.

For hypothesis 5, the relationship of change between the first and second visit of perceived health and levels of coping is significant at the $P<0.01$, and the null hypothesis of no relationship can be rejected with confidence.

And finally for hypothesis 6, the relationship of change between first and second visit of levels of coping and perception of care is not significant at the 0.05 level, and the null hypothesis is accepted.

In summary, hypothesis 1, 2, and 5 are rejected with confidence, meaning that in this study there is a significant relationship between levels of coping and certainty/uncertainty scores and perceived levels of health.

Implications for nursing practice

In coping with chronic conditions, and often there is more than one to cope with, the individual's need for certainty about his life situation, a comfortable level of perceived well-being, as well as perceived level of care are critical variables in providing nursing care. This study shows the significant relationship between these variables.

Nursing is the dynamic component for continuity of care of the elderly at home. Future research will provide more opportunities to study nursing's contribution to continuity of care. Some areas for future research include:

1. how the elderly cope with various nursing care procedures;
2. how the elderly cope in various settings, e.g. nursing homes, apartments/condominiums, senior citizen communities, and
3. how the elderly cope with other variables such as physiological functioning and psychosocial functioning.

Reference

Aiken L. (1978) Later Life. Saunders, Philadelphia.

Campbell J. (1980) The relationship of nursing and self-awareness. Advances in Nursing Science 2, 15-25.

Cowgill D.O. (1967) Toward a sociological theory of ageing based on crosscultural observations. A paper presented at the annual meeting of the Gerontological Society, St. Petersburg, Florida, November 1967.

Engel V.F. (1984) Newman's conceptual framework and the measurement of older adults' health. Advance Nursing Science 7, 24-35.

Erikson E.H. (1963) Childhood and Society 2nd edn. Norton, New York.

Frankl V.E. (1969) The Will to Meaning. New American Library, New York.

Health Care Financing Administration (1981) Long-Term Care: Background and Future Directions. Department of Health and Human Services, Washington, DC.

Mishel M.H. (1982) The measurement of uncertainty in illness. Nursing Research 3, 137-142.

Mundinger M. (1983) Home Care Controversy. Rockville, MD: Aspen Systems, Rockville, MD.

Neugarten B., Havighurst R. and Tokin S. (1961) The measurement of life satisfaction. Journal of Gerontology 16, 134-143.

Norton R.W. (1975) Measurement of ambiguity tolerance. Journal of Personal Assessment 39, 607-619.

Nursing Outlook (1972) Extending the scope of nursing practice: a report of the Secretary's Committee to Study Extend Roles of Nurses. Nursing Outlook 20, 46-52.

Pegels C. (1981) Health and Care in the Elderly. Rockville, MD: Aspen Systems, Rockville, MD.

Reed P.G. (1983) Implications of the life-span developmental framework for well being in adulthood and aging. Advances in Nursing Science 6, 18-25.

Riegel K.F. (1975) Toward a dialectical theory of development. American Psychologist 31, 689-700.

Shanas E. & Maddox G.L. (1976) Ageing, health and the organization of health resources. In Handbook of Aging and the Social Sciences (Binstock R.H. & Shanas E. eds.) Van Nostrand Reinhold, New York.

Epilogue

Our Continued Growth and Commitment

"A different world cannot be built by indifferent people."

—Thomas King

This was my father's favourite and frequently stated comment. It was always warmly said.

It has been a challenging and delightful journey. But this is NOT the end. It is only the beginning. The love and care of humanity need further research and study with a growing need for interdisciplinary leadership that possesses a creative spirit. Our professionals must choose a more collaborative and supportive path together to enrich our knowledge and skills for the humanity of professional interdisciplinary leadership and care.

NOW – it is needed. The future is in the NOW.

There are some basic principles that are essential to continue our international and national interdisciplinary growth.

Functioning principles are necessary to identify the specific area(s) for research and study. Uncertainty is no excuse for lack of courage; there will always be challenging moments.

PRINCIPLE #1

An interview of a problem(s) of concern is stated clearly following a search of the literature. Perhaps a personal (or group) survey of knowledgeable individuals/groups would also be helpful. During this process, a leader, coordinator and team members are identified and willing to assume the joy of fulfilling the study. This can be tentative throughout the literature search and survey period. Normally, the same team follows through, but at this time, the SCOPE of the study will become clear, which could influence individuals to continue after this phase or not. This is a critical moment as the strong commitment to the study is essential. Additionally, the individuals of the team must be strongly committed and respected for their decision to continue.

The success of the Study relies on this committed Research Team and the identified Team Leader.

PRINCIPLE #2

With all members of the research team assembled, the refinement of the study is established, chaired by the coordinator leader. There are then specific revisions of the refined, stated problem, and the methodology (i.e. data collection and analysis as specifically identified and discovered) and support system are identified. Frequently, a pilot study is conducted at this time to test our systems and make necessary changes as considered by the whole team, including clerical services and support system.

By this time, funding services will be clearly identified, and a grant proposal will be written that demonstrates the need for funding if additional funding is necessary. The coordinator leader will have been considering this and will review this with the team.

PRINCIPLE #3

After several weekly meetings, discussions will be held with total team – suggestions, comments, questions. The appropriate number of meetings will be determined based on the methodology.

When appropriate, analysis of the data, review of the report, further discussions and reports with interdisciplinary settings will be planned and conducted. Of course, all team members will participate and respond to members' interdisciplinary settings questions. The final report will be distributed to each interdisciplinary group.

Modifications, of course, can also be made to these basic principles, depending on the actual extent of the research study to be done. I have been told my middle name is "Let's Get Organized" King! That's true!

In Conclusion

Thank you for sharing my nursing journey with each of you – it has been a privilege.

Thank you also for your personal encouragement and caring.

I hesitate to extend the names of my many friends, supporters, and family members for fear of missing someone. Please know you are always in my prayers with my highest sincerity and love of each of you. Forever.

God bless you all.
Thank you,
Floris

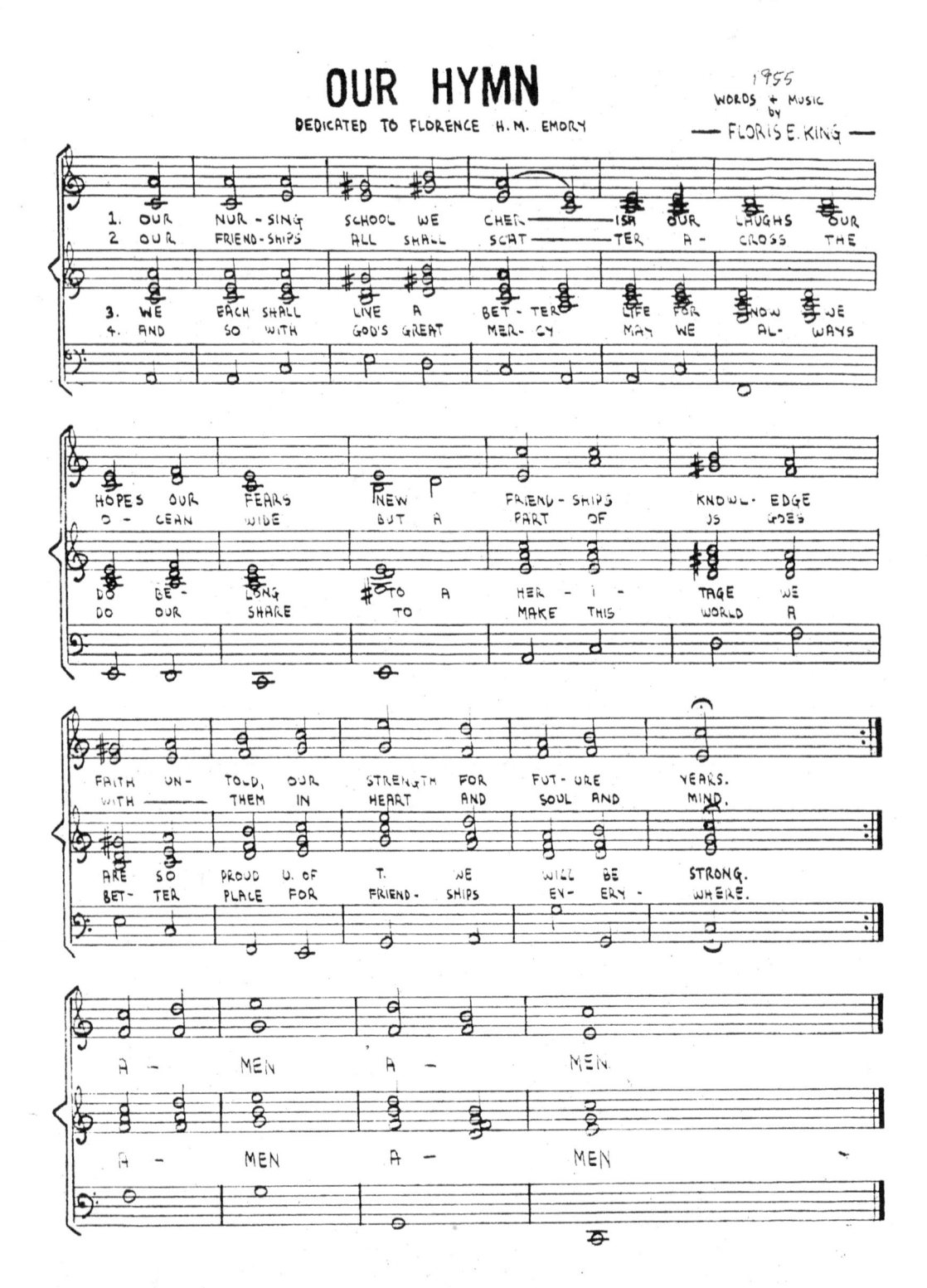

OUR HYMN

DEDICATED TO FLORENCE H.M. EMORY

1955
WORDS + MUSIC
by
— FLORIS E. KING —

1. OUR NUR-SING SCHOOL WE CHER-ISH OUR LAUGHS OUR HOPES OUR FEARS NEW FRIEND-SHIPS KNOWL-EDGE FAITH UN-TOLD, OUR STRENGTH FOR FUT-URE YEARS.
2. OUR FRIEND-SHIPS ALL SHALL SCAT-TER A-CROSS THE O-CEAN WIDE BUT A PART OF IS GOES WITH THEM IN HEART AND SOUL AND MIND.
3. WE EACH SHALL LIVE A BET-TER LIFE FOR NOW WE DO BE-LONG TO A HER-I-TAGE WE ARE SO PROUD U. OF T. WE WILL BE STRONG.
4. AND SO WITH GOD'S GREAT MER-CY MAY WE AL-WAYS DO OUR SHARE TO MAKE THIS WORLD A BET-TER PLACE FOR FRIEND-SHIPS EV-ERY-WHERE.

A-MEN A-MEN
A-MEN A-MEN